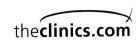

HAND CLINICS

Thumb Arthritis

GUEST EDITOR
Tamara D. Rozental, MD

August 2008 • Volume 24 • Number 3

SAUNDERS

An Imprint of Elsevier, Inc.
PHILADELPHIA   LONDON   TORONTO   MONTREAL   SYDNEY   TOKYO

W.B. SAUNDERS COMPANY

A Division of Elsevier Inc.

1600 John F. Kennedy Blvd. • Suite 1800 • Philadelphia, Pennsylvania 19103

http://www.theclinics.com

HAND CLINICS
August 2008
Editor: Debora Dellapena

Volume 24, Number 3
ISSN 0749-0712
ISBN-13: 978-1-4160-6303-2
ISBN-10: 1-4160-6303-X

Hand Clinics (ISSN 0749-0712) is published quarterly by Elsevier Inc., 360 Park Avenue South, New York, NY 10010-1710. Months of publication are February, May, August, and November. Business and Editorial Offices: 1600 John F. Kennedy Blvd., Suite 1800, Philadelphia, PA 19103-2899. Customer Service Office: 6277 Sea Harbor Drive, Orlando, FL 32887-4800. Periodicals postage paid at New York, NY, and additional mailing offices. Subscription price is $261.00 per year (U.S. individuals), $405.00 per year (U.S. institutions), $133.00 per year (US students), $297.00 per year (Canadian individuals), $454.00 per year (Canadian institutions), $164.00 (Canadian students), $333.00 per year (international individuals), $454.00 per year (international institutions), and $164.00 per year (international students). Foreign air speed delivery is included in all *Clinics* subscription prices. All prices are subject to change without notice. POSTMASTER: Send address changes to *Hand Clinics*, Elsevier Periodicals Customer Service, 6277 Sea Harbor Drive, Orlando, FL 32887-4800. Customer Service: 1-800-654-2452 (US). From outside the United States, call 1-407-563-6020. Fax: 1-407-363-9661. E-mail: JournalsCustomerService-usa@elsevier.com.

Reprints. For copies of 100 or more of articles in this publication, please contact the Commercial Reprints Department, Elsevier Inc., 360 Park Avenue South, New York, NY 10010-1710. Tel.: 212-633-3812; Fax: 212-462-1935; E-mail: reprints@elsevier.com.

Hand Clinics is covered in *MEDLINE/PubMed (Index Medicus)*, *Current Contents/Clinical Medicine*, *EMBASE/Excerpta Medica*, and *ISI/BIOMED*.

Printed in the United States of America.

GUEST EDITOR

TAMARA D. ROZENTAL, MD, Instructor in Orthopeadic Surgery, Harvard Medical School, Beth Israel Deaconess Medical Center, Boston, Massachusetts

CONTRIBUTORS

EDWARD J. ARMBRUSTER, DO, MA, Fellow in Hand, Upper Extremity and Microvascular Surgery, Department of Orthopaedics, Division of Hand and Microvascular Surgery, New Jersey Medical School, University of Medicine and Dentistry of New Jersey, Newark, New Jersey

PEDRO K. BEREDJIKLIAN, MD, Associate Professor, Department of Orthopaedic Surgery, University of Pennsylvania School of Medicine, Presbyterian Hospital, Philadelphia, Pennsylvania

DAVID J. BOZENTKA, MD, Chief of Hand Surgery, and Associate Professor of Orthopaedics, Department of Orthopaedic Surgery, University of Pennsylvania, Penn Presbyterian Medical Center, Philadelphia, Pennsylvania

LOUIS CATALANO III, MD, Assistant Clinical Professor of Orthopaedic Surgery, Columbia College of Physicians and Surgeons; Attending Physician, CV Starr Hand Surgery Center, St. Luke's—Roosevelt Hospital Center, New York, New York

ARON T. CHACKO, BS, Department of Orthopaedic Surgery, Beth Israel Deaconess Medical Center, Harvard Medical School, Boston, Massachusetts

DAMIEN I. DAVIS, MD, Resident, St. Luke's-Roosevelt Hospital Center, New York, New York

BRANDON E. EARP, MD, Department of Orthopaedic Surgery, Brigham and Women's Hospital, Boston, Massachusetts

BRIAN T. FITZGERALD, MD, Director, Division of Hand and Microvascular Surgery, Department of Orthopaedic Surgery, Naval Medical Center San Diego, San Diego, California

ERIC P. HOFMEISTER, MD, Vice Chair, Department of Orthopaedic Surgery, Division of Hand and Microvascular Surgery, Naval Medical Center San Diego, San Diego, California; Assistant Professor of Surgery, Uniformed Services University of Health Sciences, Bethesda, Maryland

JULIA A. KENNISTON, MD, Orthopaedic Resident, Department of Orthopaedic Surgery, Hospital of the University of Pennsylvania, Philadelphia, Pennsylvania

FRASER J. LEVERSEDGE, MD, Assistant Clinical Professor, Department of Orthopaedic Surgery, University of Colorado Health Sciences Center; Hand Surgery Associates, Denver, Colorado

A. LEE OSTERMAN, MD, Professor of Hand and Orthopaedic Surgery, Thomas Jefferson University Hospital, Philadelphia; and Director, The Philadelphia Hand Center, P.C., King of Prussia, Pennsylvania

MIN J. PARK, MMSc, Department of Orthopedic Surgery, Rhode Island Hospital, Warren Alpert Medical School of Brown University, Providence, Rhode Island; Department of Orthopedic Surgery, Hospital of the University of Pennsylvania, Philadelphia, Pennsylvania

TAMARA D. ROZENTAL, MD, Instructor in Orthopeadic Surgery, Harvard Medical School, Beth Israel Deaconess Medical Center, Boston, Massachusetts

EON K. SHIN, MD, Assistant Professor of Orthopaedic Surgery, Thomas Jefferson University Hospital, The Philadelphia Hand Center, P.C., Philadelphia, Pennsylvania

VIRAK TAN, MD, Program Director of the Hand, Upper Extremity and Microvascular Surgery Fellowship, and Associate Professor, Department of Orthopaedics, Division of Hand and Microvascular Surgery, New Jersey Medical School, University of Medicine and Dentistry of New Jersey, Newark, New Jersey

PETER TSAI, MD, Hand Surgery Fellow, Department of Orthopaedic Surgery, University of Pennsylvania School of Medicine, Presbyterian Hospital, Philadelphia, Pennsylvania

JENNIFER MORIATIS WOLF, MD, Assistant Professor, Department of Orthopaedics, University of Colorado Denver School of Medicine, Aurora, Colorado

JEFFREY YAO, MD, Robert A. Chase Hand and Upper Limb Center, Department of Orthopedic Surgery, Stanford University Hospitals and Clinics, Palo Alto, California

CONTENTS

population. Because of its high prevalence, the management of the condition has been a popular topic among hand surgeons and therapists worldwide. There are many decisions to consider when devising the appropriate treatment plan for each patient. In particular, early stages of thumb CMC joint arthritis may be treated nonoperatively or with less invasive surgical techniques to relieve symptoms, restore function and strength, stop the progression of the disease, and even potentially reverse the process. This article explores treatment options at the disposal of primary care physicians and hand surgeons for early thumb CMC arthritis.

carpometacarpal arthritis. For isolated trapeziometacarpal arthritis, arthrodesis is a viable option to create a pain free, strong, and stable thumb.

FORTHCOMING ISSUES

RECENT ISSUES

Preface

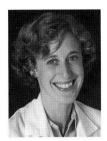

Tamara D. Rozental, MD
Guest Editor

With an aging population, arthritis is becoming a leading source of disability in our society. In particular, arthritis of the thumb (with ensuing pain and loss of motion) causes significant functional limitations in an increasingly active patient population. Thus, it is essential for upper extremity surgeons to develop and maintain detailed knowledge of the anatomy, clinical presentation, and available treatment options for this common condition. This issue of *Hand Clinics* attempts to provide a review of the pathoanatomy, physical examination, and imaging options available for the diagnosis of thumb arthritis. Subsequently, treatment options for early and advanced disease are explored in greater depth. Some of the described procedures have been employed for several decades; others are more recent and gaining in popularity. I am indebted to the talented group of individuals who contributed articles to this publication. Their time, energy, and enthusiasm generated what I consider to be a useful tool for any hand surgeon's practice.

Tamara D. Rozental, MD
Harvard Medical School
Beth Israel Deaconess Medical Center
330 Brookline Avenue, Stoneman 10
Boston, MA 02215, USA

E-mail address: trozenta@bidmc.harvard.edu

0749-0712/08/$ - see front matter © 2008 Elsevier Inc. All rights reserved.
doi:10.1016/j.hcl.2008.03.009

ELSEVIER
SAUNDERS

Hand Clin 24 (2008) 219–229

HAND
CLINICS

Anatomy and Pathomechanics of the Thumb

Fraser J. Leversedge, MD[a,b,*]

[a]*Department of Orthopaedic Surgery, University of Colorado Health Sciences Center,*
2535 South Downing, Suite 500, Denver, CO 80210, USA
[b]*Hand Surgery Associates, 2535 South Downing, Suite 500, Denver, CO 80210, USA*

Thumb anatomy

Evolution of thumb anatomy

Human evolution has been distinguished, in part, by the development of the prehensile thumb, facilitating dexterous and fine motor pinch and grasp. In contrast to simian ancestors whose thumb motion was limited to a flexion-extension arc in the plane of the palm [1], the human thumb has evolved through a relative loss of stability, in the process gaining prehension, opposition, and circumduction via the development of a bicon-cave-convex trapeziometacarpal (TM) saddle joint and the actions of associated intrinsic and extrinsic musculotendinous structures. The ability for the specialized thumb to rotate and to oppose the fingers provides a functional advantage and was observed by Aristotle [2]:

The joints, moreover, of the fingers are well constructed for prehension and for pressure. One of these also, and this not long like the rest but short and thick, is placed laterally. For were it not placed all prehension would be as impossible, as were there no hand at all. For the pressure of this digit is applied from below upwards, while the rest act from above downwards; an arrangement which is essential, if the grasp is to be firm and hold like a tight clamp. As for the shortness of this digit, the object is to increase its strength, so that it may be able, through but one, to counterbalance its more numerous opponents.

Understanding the pathophysiology of the thumb "basal joint" requires a sound appreciation

---

* Hand Surgery Associates, 2535 South Downing, Suite 500, Denver, CO 80210.

E-mail address: fraserjl@comcast.net

for its complex anatomy and its kinematics. The pantrapezial basal joint involves directly the five articulations of the TM, scaphotrapezial, scapho-trapezoidal, trapezium-index metacarpal, and trapezium-trapezoid joints; also, the indirect influences of the thumb metacarpophalangeal (MCP) joint and interphalangeal (IP) joint may contribute to alterations in basal joint mechanics. Therefore, it is imperative that treatment decisions for basal joint pathology consider a global assessment of the pathoanatomy and pathomechanics of each articulation.

Trapeziometacarpal joint

The thumb TM joint, or carpometacarpal (CMC) joint, is a biconcave-convex or reciprocal saddle joint. The articular structure provides little inherent constraint for joint stability and, therefore, relies on the 16 described ligaments that stabilize the TM joint and the trapezium [3,4]. The axis of the thumb at the TM joint rests in a pronated position, flexed approximately 80° relative to the plane of the metacarpals of the fingers [5,6]. This optimizes thumb positioning for opposition to the tips of the fingers for prehensile activities.

Measurement of the curved articular dimensions of the TM joint have been reported by Bettinger and Berger [7]. The midsagittal (dorsal-volar direction) diameter of the thumb metacarpal base is 16.03 ± 1.27 mm and the midsagittal diameter of the trapezium is 11.96 ± 1.32 mm. This discrepancy in the diameters of the articulating surfaces is approximately 34%; the increased diameter of the thumb metacarpal base relative to the trapezial joint surface has implications for joint stability through contributions of the stabilizing ligaments of the TM joint relative to thumb position [5]. Fig. 1 depicts the application of

0749-0712/08/$ - see front matter © 2008 Elsevier Inc. All rights reserved.
doi:10.1016/j.hcl.2008.03.010

hand.theclinics.com

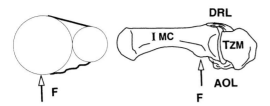

Fig. 1. Ligamentous restraint of the TM joint to a dor-sally directed force on the first metacarpal and two spheres connected by two cords representing the relative midsagittal diameters of the I metacarpal and trapezium. The DRL tightens and the AOL becomes lax on applica-tion of this force vector. This is because the midsagittal diameter of the first metacarpal is greater than the mid-sagittal diameter of the trapezium. (*Reprinted from* Bet-tinger PC, Berger RA. Functional ligamentous anatomy of the trapezium and trapeziometacarpal joint [gross and arthroscopic]. Hand Clin 2001;17:166; with permission.)

a dorsally directed force on the TM joint and demonstrates how the size discrepancy of the thumb metacarpal base and trapezium promotes tightening of the dorsoradial ligament (DRL) to stabilize the TM joint while the anterior oblique ligament (AOL) becomes lax. Kuczynski [8] has demonstrated that the architecture of the trapezial joint surface may promote pronation of the thumb metacarpal, although other factors may contribute to thumb metacarpal pronation during the initiation of opposition. A force nucleus con-cept has been proposed by Zancolli [9], whereby a force couple is developed through muscle activ-ity and passive ligament tension; others have iden-tified the deep anterior oblique ligament (dAOL) as a potential pivot point for the TM joint pas-sively guiding the joint into pronation as the in-trinsic motor function actively pulls the thumb into abduction and flexion [4,10].

Anatomic dissections of the stabilizing liga-ments of the thumb TM joint have demonstrated a complex arrangement of intricate constraints supporting the TM joint and the great forces imparted to the joint with pinch and grasp activity. These observations are complimented through the use of arthroscopic evaluation; the TM ligaments may be well visualized from an undisturbed intra-articular perspective. Original anatomic study of the TM joint by Weitbrecht [11] has been further clarified by contributions from various investigators [5,6,12–19], most recently Bettinger and colleagues [4]. Previously, Bettinger and Berger [7] have defined the anatomic orienta-tion of the thumb and their summary for descrip-tive purposes is used in this article. The term,

dorsal, refers to that which lies within the plane of the thumbnail, and the terms, volar and pal-mar, refer to that within the plane of the pulp. The terms, radial and ulnar, describe the respec-tive sides of the thumb when the thumbnail is parallel to the fingernails; the thumb is in a posi-tion of supination and radial abduction relative to the fixed axis of the hand. The 16 ligaments as described by Bettinger and colleagues [4] and Bettinger and Berger [7] are reviewed.

Superior anterior oblique ligament

Immediately deep to the thenar musculature, which overlies the volar aspect of the TM joint and is superficial to the dAOL, the superior anterior oblique ligament (SAOL) capsular liga-ment has been described by Pieron [6] as running in a "curtain-like" fashion. Its relative laxity is observed to permit essential joint mobility, partic-ularly that of pronation required for opposition [4,18]. The SAOL is lax throughout most of the TM range of motion except for becoming taut at the extremes of thumb pronation and extension. The ligament originates 0.5 mm proximal to the articular surface at the volar tubercle of the trape-zium and inserts broadly over the volar ulnar tubercle of the thumb metacarpal base, 2 mm dis-tal to the volar styloid process.

Deep anterior oblique ligament
(palmar beak ligament)

The dAOL is an intra-articular ligament that lies deep to the SAOL, originating from the volar central apex of the trapezium, ulnar to the ulnar edge of the trapezial ridge, and inserting into the articular margin ulnar to the volar styloid process (volar beak) of the thumb metacarpal base. The dAOL becomes taut with increasing thumb ab-duction, pronation, and extension. Its fiber orien-tation resists ulnar subluxation of the thumb metacarpal base with progressive abduction load-ing of the thumb and prevents volar subluxation of the TM joint [19,20]. The static constraint of the dAOL and its intra-articular location at the volar-ulnar corner of the joint creates a pivot point around which the thumb metacarpal rotates into pronation with applied intrinsic forces of flex-ion and abduction.

Dorsoradial ligament

The wide, fan-shaped DRL is a short capsular ligament that arises from the dorsoradial tubercle of the trapezium and has a broad insertion into the dorsal base of the thumb metacarpal. Although there have been discrepancies in identifying the contributions of the DRL to TM joint stability [18,19,21–23], Bettinger and colleagues [4] demonstrated that the DRL tightens to resist a dorsal or dorsoradial subluxing force in all joint positions except for TM joint extension and that it likely is a primary stabilizer resisting dorsal and dorsoradial forces. In all joint positions, the DRL tightens with supination of the thumb, and in TM joint flexion the DRL tightens with thumb pronation. In a serial sectioning study assessing the dorsal stabilizers of the TM joint, Van Brenk and colleagues [23] reported that insufficiency of the DRL resulted in the greatest dorsoradial subluxation. Ligament reconstruction, described by Eaton and Littler, which uses a dorsal-radial drill hole in the thumb metacarpal base, effectively recreates the DRL through the dorsal transfer and stabilization of the flexor carpi ulnaris (FCR) in this position [7].

Posterior oblique ligament

The posterior oblique ligament (POL) is a capsular ligament that originates on the dorsal-ulnar aspect of the trapezium, immediately ulnar to the DRL, and runs obliquely to insert at the dorsal-ulnar aspect of the thumb metacarpal and the palmar-ulnar tubercle, adjacent to the intermetacarpal ligament (IML). The POL tightens with thumb abduction, opposition, and supination and the POL prevents ulnar translation of the thumb metacarpal base during opposition and abduction.

Ulnar collateral ligament

The ulnar collateral ligament (UCL) is an extracapsular ligament that takes it origin from the distal margin of the transverse carpal ligament (TCL) and the trapezial ridge and inserts onto the palmar-ulnar tubercle of the thumb metacarpal adjacent to the IML. The UCL insertion is superficial and ulnar to the SAOL. The UCL is taut with progressive thumb extension, abduction, and pronation. It acts with the SAOL and dAOL to prevent volar subluxation of the thumb metacarpal base.

Intermetacarpal ligament

The extracapsular IML originates radial to the extensor carpi radialis longus (ECRL) insertion at the dorsal base of the index metacarpal and inserts onto the palmar-ulnar tubercle of the thumb metacarpal base adjacent to the POL and UCL. There are variable descriptions of the IML, including a dorsal IML and a Y-shaped ligament morphology. The IML is taut with thumb abduction, opposition, and supination and it resists radial and volar translation of the metacarpal base.

Dorsal intermetacarpal ligament

The extracapsular dorsal IML (DIML) originates from the dorsoradial tubercle of the index metacarpal base, distal and superficial to the ECRL insertion, and inserts onto the dorsal-ulnar margin of the thumb metacarpal base. Occasionally, the DIML insertion may have two limbs, similar to that of a "Y," both of which insert into the thumb metacarpal. The DIML is tight with thumb pronation and also with dorsal and radial translation of the thumb metacarpal base. The DIML and the IM may provide contributing support to prevent proximal migration of the thumb metacarpal base after trapeziectomy and ligament reconstruction and tendon interposition arthroplasty [7].

Dorsal trapeziotrapezoid ligament

The dorsal trapeziotrapezoid (DTT) ligament is a capsular ligament that originates from the proximal half of the dorsal-ulnar margin of the trapezium and inserts onto the proximal half of the dorsal-radial margin of the trapezoid. The DTT stabilizes the trapeziotrapezoid joint and resists extension, radial deviation, and pronation of the trapezium.

Volar trapeziotrapezoid ligament

The volar trapeziotrapezoid (VTT) is a capsular ligament that originates from the volar-ulnar tubercle of the trapezium and inserts onto the volar-radial corner of the trapezoid. Its insertion is deep to the origin of the trapezio-capitate (T-C) ligament and the two ligaments typically are separated by a fibrofatty synovial tissue. The VTT and the DTT stabilize the trapeziotrapezoid joint; the VTT resists trapezial supination.

Dorsal trapezio-II metacarpal ligament

This capsular ligament (dorsal trapezio-II metacarpal ligament [DT-II MC]) originates at the dorsal-ulnar tubercle of the trapezium runs obliquely to insert onto the dorsal-ulnar margin of the index metacarpal base, deep to the insertion of the ECRL tendon. It is suggested that the DT-II MC functions as an effective tension band to resist cantilever bending forces (extension and radial translation) acting on the trapezium [24].

Volar trapezio-II metacarpal ligament

The volar trapezio-II metacarpal (VT-II MC) ligament arises from the volar-ulnar aspect of the trapezium and inserts into the volar-radial corner of the index metacarpal. This capsular ligament is similar in its function to that of the DT-II MC ligament in that it resists cantilever bending of the trapezium [24]. The VT-II MC also resists supination of the trapezium.

Trapezio-III metacarpal ligament

The trapezio-III metacarpal (T-III MC) ligament originates superficial and proximal to the VT-II MC ligament at the volar-ulnar corner of the trapezium and traverses a small groove formed by the volar tubercle of the index metacarpal to insert into the volar-radial corner of the long finger metacarpal. The T-III MC ligament is extracapsular and resists supination and cantilever bending of the trapezium.

Transverse carpal ligament

The TCL is an extracapsular ligament that resists extension, radial deviation, and supination of the trapezium through its stabilizing attachments from the hook of the hamate and pisiform (origin) to its insertion at the scaphoid and volar ridge of the trapezium.

Trapezio-capitate ligament

The T-C ligament overlies and is more substantial than the VTT ligament, traversing from its origin at the volar-ulnar corner of the proximal

half trapezium to insert into the distal half of the volar-radial margin of the capitate. The extracapsular T-C ligament forms part of the floor of the FCR tunnel and, similar to the VTT, stabilizes the trapezium from cantilever bending forces and supination.

Volar scaphotrapezial ligament

The capsular volar scaphotrapezial (VST) ligament originates from the scaphoid tuberosity and inserts into the proximal quarter of the volar trapezium. The VST is taut with the trapezium in extension or with progressive rotation of the trapezium (pronation or supination).

Radial scaphotrapezial ligament

This capsular ligament originates from the scaphoid tuberosity and inserts into the radial margin of the trapezial ridge and radial aspect of the trapezium. The radial scaphotrapezial (RST) ligament resists progressive rotation of the trapezium (pronation or supination) (Figs. 2–7).

The flexion-extension axis of the TM joint is oriented out of the plane of the palm and, relative to the axis of the long finger metacarpal, is positioned at approximately 40° of abduction, 50° of flexion, and 80° of pronation [25]. Cooney and Chao [26] reported that TM joint range of motion in the flexion-extension plane is

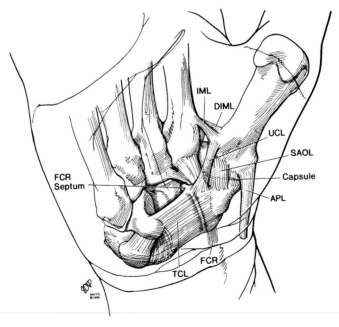

Fig. 2. Superficial volar ligaments of the trapezium and TM joint. (*Courtesy of* the Mayo Foundation, Rochester, MN; with permission.)

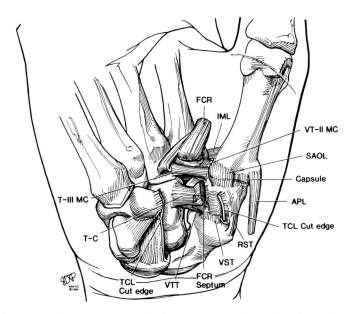

Fig. 3. Deep volar ligaments of the trapezium and TM joint. Note the FCR is reflected distally, and the TCL has been excised. (*Courtesy of* the Mayo Foundation, Rochester, MN; with permission.)

$53° \pm 11°$ and is $42° \pm 4°$ in the plane of abduction-adduction.

Metacarpophalangeal joint

The thumb MCP joint resembles a ball-and-socket joint with 3° of freedom. Motion occurs in the flexion-extension plane primarily; however, there is motion in the abduction-adduction plane limited by the soft tissue constraints and a limited degree of rotation occurring through the joint [27]. The thumb metacarpal head typically is a single, broad condyle rounded in 90% and flattened in 10% of the population. The joint is stabilized primarily by the radial (RCL) collateral ligament, the UCL, and the thick, fibrocartilage volar plate [28]. The collateral ligaments are comprised of the proper and accessory collateral ligaments; the proper collateral ligament originates from the lateral and dorsal margin of the metacarpal head and runs obliquely to insert into the volar-ulnar base of the proximal phalanx. The origin of the accessory collateral ligament is proximal and volar to that of the proper collateral ligament and it runs obliquely to insert into the volar plate (Fig. 8). The volar plate resists MCP joint hyperextension. It originates at the volar neck of the metacarpal and inserts volarly into the base of the proximal phalanx. The volar plate contains

the sesamoids; the radial sesamoid is a site of insertion for the flexor pollicis brevis (FPB). Dorsally, the MCP joint capsule inserts into the dorsal base of the proximal phalanx and, along with the thumb sagittal band, provides minimal indirect stability to the MCP joint.

The joint is dynamically stabilized during pinch and grasp activity through the actions of the abductor pollicis brevis (APB), adductor pollicis (ADD), FPB, and extensor pollicis brevis (EPB) muscles (Figs. 9–12) [29]. The pertinent anatomic relationships of these musculotendinous units are reviewed.

Interphalangeal joint

The thumb IP joint is stabilized by the volar plate, the collateral ligaments, and the insertions of the flexor pollicis longus (FPL) tendon and the extensor pollicis longus (EPL) tendon at the volar base and dorsal base of the distal phalanx, respectively [29]. The head of the proximal phalanx includes two condyles separated by an intercondylar notch, which provides some relative stability through its articulation with the median ridge of the base of the distal phalanx similar to that of the proximal IP joint of the finger. Normal IP joint range of motion is from approximately 20° of extension beyond neutral through 75° to

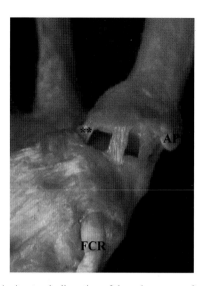

Fig. 4. Anatomic dissection of the volar aspect of a right thumb TM joint. The FCR tendon angles dorsally at the trapezial groove to insert at the volar base of the index metacarpal. The TCL is superficial to the FCR tendon. The dAOL (**), or volar beak ligament, is the primary stabilizer of the thumb TM joint. The intra-articular dDAOL originates at the volar-ulnar corner of the thumb metacarpal base and inserts into the volar tubercle of the trapezium. In this dissection, the superficial anterior oblique ligament and TM joint capsule has been removed, with a portion of the SAOL preserved and visualized at the center of the joint. The APL tendon (AP) inserts into the radial base of the thumb metacarpal (cut). (*Courtesy of* F. J. Leversedge, MD, Denver, CO; and C. A. Goldfarb, MD, St. Louis, MO; and M. I. Boyer, MD, St. Louis, MO. Copyright ©2008; used with permission.)

80° of flexion [30]. Joint extension may be powered through the actions of the EPL, APB, ADD, and FPB, whereas the FPL is the exclusive flexor of the IP joint.

Musculotendinous anatomy

Thumb motion is coordinated through the influences of extrinsic and extrinsic musculature. These motor units may act as dynamic stabilizers of the thumb, facilitating pinch and grasp function [29]. Variations in anatomy, by injury or as congenital anomaly, may influence the transmission of force through the thumb. Neurologic deficit may directly alter the biomechanics of the thumb, such as from a motor imbalance after ulnar nerve injury and subsequent intrinsic motor palsy.

Extrinsic musculotendinous anatomy influencing thumb motion and stability includes the abductor pollicis longus (APL), EPL, extensor pollicis bravis (EPB), and FPL tendons.

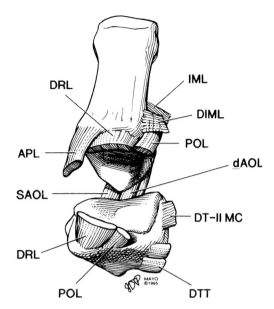

Fig. 5. The TM joint has been hinged open from the dorsum to reveal the dAOL (beak ligament) lying within the joint just ulnar to the volar tubercle of the metacarpal. (*Courtesy of* the Mayo Foundation, Rochester, MN; with permission.)

The APL originates from the dorsal surface of the radius, traveling distally within the first extensor compartment, palmar to the EPB tendon, to insert into the thumb metacarpal base, the trapezium, and the thenar musculature (variable: opponens ± APB). The APL may have one or multiple tendon slips (two is most common) [31,32]. The APL is innervated by the posterior interosseous nerve and functions to primarily extend and mildly abduct the thumb metacarpal.

The EPB originates from the interosseous membrane of the forearm and occasionally from the dorsal surface of the radius and runs within the first extensor compartment as one tendon slip, although it may run within its own subcompartment 30% of the time [32]. The EPB tendon typically inserts into the base of the proximal phalanx, radial to the distally directed EPL tendon, although variations of its insertion, including that into the extensor hood, are described [33]. The EPB is innervated by the posterior interosseous nerve and functions to extend the MCP joint of the thumb and may contribute to IP joint extension but not to IP joint hyperextension.

The EPL originates from the ulna and runs distally, angling 45° radially at Lister's tubercle, to insert into the dorsal base of the thumb distal

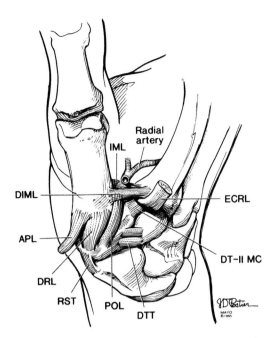

Fig. 6. DRLs of the trapezium and TM joint. Note the ECRL tendon has been reflected distally. (*Courtesy of the Mayo Foundation, Rochester, MN; with permission.*)

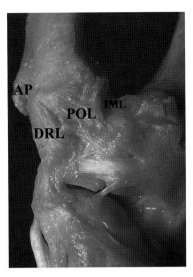

Fig. 7. The dorsal aspect of the thumb TM joint. The AP tendon has been cut from its insertion into the radial base of the thumb metacarpal. The DRL originates at the dorsoradial tubercle of the trapezium and inserts onto the dorsal base of the thumb metacarpal. The POL originates on the dorsal-ulnar aspect of the trapezium, immediately ulnar to the DRL, and runs obliquely to insert at the dorsal-ulnar aspect of the thumb metacarpal and the palmar-ulnar tubercle, adjacent to the IML. The first IML originates at the dorsal base of the index metacarpal and inserts onto the palmar-ulnar tubercle of the thumb metacarpal base. (*Courtesy of* F. J. Leversedge, MD, Denver, CO; and C. A. Goldfarb, MD, St. Louis, MO; and M. I. Boyer, MD, St. Louis, MO. Copyright ©2008; used with permission.)

phalanx. It is innervated by the posterior interosseous nerve and functions to extend the thumb IP joint and to adduct the thumb.

The FPL originates from the anterior surface of the radius and interosseous membrane and runs distally as a deep forearm flexor to insert into the volar base of the thumb distal phalanx. The FPL may have an accessory head, originating from the proximal ulna or medial epicondyle (Gantzer's muscle). A tendinous interconnection (Linburg-Comstock anomaly) between the index FDP and FPL may be present in the forearm (25%–30% unilateral, 5%–15% bilateral), resulting in an interdependence of tendon excursion between the two tendons [34]. Innervated by the anterior interosseous nerve, the FPL flexes the thumb IP joint.

Intrinsic musculotendinous anatomy influencing thumb function includes the APB, ADD, FPB, and opponens pollicis (OP) [35–37].

The APB originates from the TCL, FCR tendon sheath, trapezium, and scaphoid and inserts into the radial base of the proximal phalanx, the MCP joint capsule, and the radial sesamoid. It is innervated by the median nerve (95%) or ulnar nerve (2.5%), or by dual median and ulnar innervation (2.5%). The APB functions to abduct and flex the thumb metacarpal, to

extend the thumb IP joint, and to ulnarly deviate the MCP joint.

The ADD originates from the long finger metacarpal and inserts into the ulnar base of the proximal phalanx, the dorsal-extensor apparatus, and the ulnar sesamoid. It is innervated by the ulnar nerve. The ADD functions to adduct the thumb metacarpal and to extend the thumb IP joint.

The FPB originates from the TCL and inserts into the MCP joint capsule and into the radial sesamoid. The superficial head is innervated by the median nerve and the deep head is innervated by the ulnar nerve. The FPB functions to flex the thumb MCP joint and the proximal phalanx, to extend the IP joint, and to pronate the thumb.

The OP originates from the TCL, the trapezium, and the thumb CMC joint capsule and inserts into the distal volar-radial thumb metacarpal. It is innervated by the median nerve (83%) or ulnar nerve (10%) or by dual median and ulnar

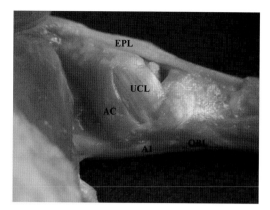

Fig. 8. The adductor aponeurosis has been removed (see Fig. 9) in this anatomic dissection, revealing the ulnar aspect of the thumb MCP joint. The UCL and the AC originate at the dorsal-ulnar margin of the head of the metacarpal; the UCL inserts into the ulnar base of the proximal phalanx and the AC inserts into the volar plate of the MCP joint. The EPL is dorsal to the MCP joint and the A1 and oblique (OBL) pulleys of the flexor sheath are noted volar to the MCP joint and the proximal phalanx. (*Courtesy of* F. J. Leversedge, MD, Denver, CO; and C. A. Goldfarb, MD, St. Louis, MO; and M. I. Boyer, MD, St. Louis, MO. Copyright ©2008; used with permission.)

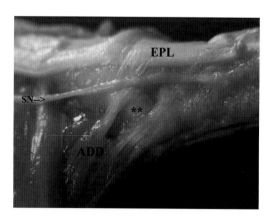

Fig. 9. Anatomic dissection of the ulnar aspect of the thumb MCP joint demonstrating the insertion of the ADD into the dorsal apparatus (stabilizing retinaculum of the EPL), the ulnar sesamoid of the thumb, and the ulnar base of the proximal phalanx. Often, there are multiple sensory nerve branches (sn) traversing the ulnar margin of the MP joint region. The UCL of the thumb MP joint is identified deep to the adductor aponeurosis (**). (*Courtesy of* F. J. Leversedge, MD, Denver, CO; and C. A. Goldfarb, MD, St. Louis, MO; and M. I. Boyer, MD, St. Louis, MO. Copyright ©2008; used with permission.)

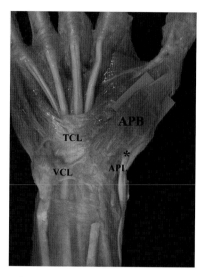

Fig. 10. Anatomic dissection of the APB and its relationships. The APB originates from the TCL and inserts into the radial base of the thumb proximal phalanx, the thumb MP joint capsule, and the radial sesamoid of the thumb. The extrinsic APL is seen inserting, in part, into the APB muscle (*). The FPB and ADD muscles are dorsal to the APB. VCL, volar carpal ligament. (*Courtesy of* F. J. Leversedge, MD, Denver, CO; and C. A. Goldfarb, MD, St. Louis, MO; and M. I. Boyer, MD, St. Louis, MO. Copyright ©2008; used with permission.)

innervation (7%). The OP functions to flex and pronate the thumb metacarpal.

Pathomechanics of the thumb

Clinical pathology at the thumb basal joint involves a complex interplay of biochemical and biomechanical factors [38,39]. The large compressive loads and shear forces acting on the articular surface may contribute to hyalaine cartilage degeneration in the presence of a biochemical environment, which promotes proteoglycan matrix catabolism, production of chondrocyte-derived degradative enzymes, and dehydration of the cartilage extracellular matrix [39]. Hormonal influences on the physiology of cartilaginous and collagenous tissues may play a central role in the recognized gender predisposition for osteoarthritis.

Eaton and Littler observed that the dorsoradial facet of the TM joint often was the first site of articular wear and hypothesized that compressive loading from the adjacent insertion of the APL during thumb extension and palmar abduction contributed to this deterioration [40–42]. Subsequent anatomic and pathologic study of

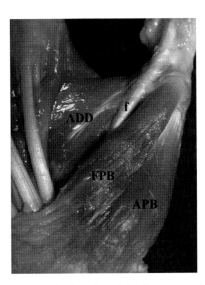

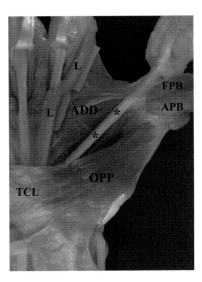

Fig. 11. Anatomic dissection of the thenar musculature. The APB and the FPB muscles originate from the TCL; the FPB origin is more distal than that of the APB. The FPL tendon (f) emerges from the interval between the deeper ADD muscle and the FPB/APB. (*Courtesy of* F. J. Leversedge, MD, Denver, CO; and C. A. Goldfarb, MD, St. Louis, MO; and M. I. Boyer, MD, St. Louis, MO. Copyright ©2008; used with permission.)

Fig. 12. Palmar view of the deep thenar musculature relationships after distal reflection of the FPB and APB muscles. The opponens pollicis (OPP) originates from the TCL, the trapezium, and the thumb CMC joint capsule and it inserts into the volar-radial distal thumb metacarpal. The OPP muscle acts to flex and pronate the thumb metacarpal. The FPL tendon (*) is seen to emerge from the carpal canal to run radially on the palmar surface of the ADD, deep to the OPP muscle. The lumbrical muscle to the index finger (L) is identified at its origin along the radial and volar margins of the flexor digitorum profundus tendon to the index finger. (*Courtesy of* F. J. Leversedge, MD, Denver, CO; and C. A. Goldfarb, MD, St. Louis, MO; and M. I. Boyer, MD, St. Louis, MO. Copyright ©2008; used with permission.)

the aging TM joint by Pellegrini [10,18] demonstrated patterns of articular degeneration and supported previous empiric evidence that correlated ligamentous laxity with progressive articular wear. Study of human cadaveric specimens demonstrated a direct correlation between the status of the articular surfaces and the integrity of the beak ligament. Although the dorsal compartment of the TM joint was found to have greater chondromalacic change, this often was the site of the only remaining articular cartilage in the severely affected osteoarthritic joint. In contrast, the palmar surfaces of the TM joint were found "polished to eburnated bone." In all cases of articular eburnation, complete detachment of the palmar beak ligament was identified. Articular wear was noted to occur earliest at the palmar perimeter of the TM joint, progressing dorsally with advanced disease.

Biochemical evaluation of hyaline cartilage harvested from the palmar margins of osteoarthritic TM joints demonstrated a preferential loss of glycosaminoglycan from the extracellular matrix, despite a relative preservation of the collagen structural matrix [43]. This selective degradation of glycosaminoglycan supports the theory of a biochemical contribution to the biomechanical

failure of hyaline cartilage, as demonstrated by scanning electron microscopy study of the arthritic TM articular surface, which has revealed a delamination of the superficial cartilage layer in the palmar joint contact areas [38].

Biomechanical studies of force transmission through the thumb axis demonstrated that a pinch force of 1 kg at the thumb tip was amplified to 3.68 kg at the IP joint, 6.61 kg at the MCP joint, and up to 13.42 kg at the TM joint. Applied force to the thumb during grasping activity can approach 20 kg [26]. Cantilever bending loads produce dorsoradial-directed force at the thumb metacarpal base, resulting in translational or shear forces and associated cartilage erosion at the TM joint. Measurement of joint contact pressure patterns in a cadaver model have demonstrated higher loading forces at the palmar surfaces of the TM joint, correlating to the surgical and cadaveric findings of eburnated articular surfaces at this location with progressive osteoarthritis, and contact forces have been observed to be greater with the joint in flexion [44–46].

Alterations in joint contact forces may occur after joint injury, surgical extension osteotomy of the thumb metacarpal, and changes in neuromuscular balance affecting the thumb, and contact stresses may be influenced by changes in force vectors by differential positioning of the thumb MCP and IP joints. Injury to the dAOL, or beak ligament, similar to the effect of attritional wear, is analogous to Bennett's-type fracture, involving a discontinuity of the ligament's attachment to the thumb metacarpal base. These injuries result in a destabilization of the thumb base and the potential development of osteoarthritic change in the involved TM joint [47,48]. In similar fashion, ligamentous laxity or hypermobility of the thumb basal joint is described as a precursor to the development of osteoarthritis of the TM joint and may be more prevalent in women [40,41,49,50]. Joint contact forces may be influenced surgically, such as with an extension osteotomy of the thumb metacarpal base. Recognition of the pathomechanics of TM joint degeneration facilitates the consideration of this treatment for selected patients who may benefit from transferring load away from the degenerative palmar articular surface to the less affected dorsal joint [51–53]. Load transfer can occur clinically, through effective modifications of pinch activity. Although MCP joint hyperextension deformity is believed a compensatory functional mechanism for progressive loss of motion at the TM joint, forces transmitted by pinch through a hyperextended MCP joint concentrate the load at the palmar TM joint compartment, thereby accelerating the disease process. Therefore, patients who have compensatory hyperextension or those patients who have extension laxity at the MCP joint without existing osteoarthritis may be predisposed for progressive basal joint arthritis, and strategies should be considered for minimizing articular wear [54].

Summary

The prehensile thumb provides the human mind an outlet for coordinated activity through its fine motions of prehension, opposition, and circumduction. A comprehensive understanding of the anatomy and biomechanics of the thumb provides a foundation on which functional disorders may be recognized and effectively treated.

References

[1] Pellegrini VD Jr. The ABJS 2005 Nicolas Andry Award: osteoarthritis and injury at the base of the human thumb: survival of the fittest? Clin Orthop Relat Res 2005;438:266–76.
[2] Smith JA, Ross WD, editors. The works of Aristotle (translated into English). Book IV, vol. V. Ogle W. De partibus animalium. Oxford: Clarendon Press; 1956. p. 686–7.
[3] Berger RA. A technique for arthroscopic evaluation of the first carpometacarpal joint. J Hand Surg [Am] 1997;22:1077–80.
[4] Bettinger PC, Linscheid RL, Berger RA. An anatomic study of the stabilizing ligaments of the trapezium and trapeziometacarpal joint. J Hand Surg [Am] 1999;24:786–98.
[5] Napier JR. The form and function of the carpometacarpal joint of the thumb. J Anat 1955;89:362–9.
[6] Pieron AP. The mechanism of the first carpometacarpal joint: an anatomical and mechanical analysis. Acta Orthop Scand Suppl 1973;148:1–104.
[7] Bettinger PC, Berger RA. Functional ligamentous anatomy of the trapezium and trapeziometacarpal joint (gross and arthroscopic). Hand Clin 2001;17:151–68.
[8] Kuczynski K. Carpometacarpal joint of the human thumb. J Anat 1974;118:119.
[9] Zancolli E. Structural and dynamic bases of hand surgery. 2nd edition. Philadelphia: JB Lippincott; 1979. p. 15–23.
[10] Pellegrini VD Jr. Osteoarthritis of the trapeziometacarpal joint: the pathophysiology of articular cartilage degeneration. II. Articular wear patterns in the osteoarthritic joint. J Hand Surg [Am] 1991;16:975–82.
[11] Weitbrecht J. Syndesmology (1742). Philadelphia: JB Saunders; 1969.
[12] Rouviere H. Anatomie humaine descriptive et topographique. Tome 2. Membres, systeme nerveux central. Paris: Masson; 1924.
[13] Haines R. The mechanism of rotation of the first carpo-metacarpal joint. J Anat 1944;78:44–6.
[14] Lanz TV, Wchsmuth W. Praktiche anatomie; ein lehr—und helfsbuch der anatomischen grundlagen arzlichen Handelns. Berlin: Springer-Verlag; 1959. p. 261.
[15] Kaplan E. Functional and surgical anatomy of the hand. 2nd edition. Philadelphia: JB Lippincott; 1965.
[16] De la Caffiniere JY. L'articulation trapezo-metacarpienne approche bio-mecanique et appareil ligamentaire. Arch Anat Pathol 1970;18:277–84.
[17] Drewniany J, Palmer A, Flatt A. The scaphotrapezial ligament complex: an anatomic and biomechanical study. J Hand Surg [Am] 1985;10:492–8.
[18] Pellegrini VD Jr. Osteoarthritis of the trapeziometacarpal joint: the pathophysiology of articular cartilage degeneration. I. Anatomy and pathology of the aging joint. J Hand Surg [Am] 1991;16:967–74.

[19] Imaeda T, An K, Cooney W, et al. Anatomy of trapeziometacarpal ligaments. J Hand Surg [Am] 1993;18:226–31.

[20] Niebur G, Imeada T, An K-N. Ligament activity of the first carpometacarpal joint. In: Langrana N, Friedman M, Good E, editors. Bioengineering conference. Colorado (AZ): American Society of Mechanical Engineers; 1993. p. 580–3.

[21] Pagalidis T, Kuczynski K, Lamb DW. Ligamentous stability of the base of the thumb. Hand 1981;13:29–35.

[22] Strauch R, Behrman M, Rosenwasser M. Acute dislocations of the carpometacarpal joint of the thumb: an anatomic and cadaver study. J Hand Surg [Am] 1994;19:93–8.

[23] Van Brenk B, Richards RR, Mackay MB, et al. A biomechanical assessment of ligaments preventing dorsoradial subluxation of the trapeziometacarpal joint. J Hand Surg [Am] 1998;23:607–11.

[24] Linscheid R. The thumb axis joints: a biomechanical model. In: Strickland JE, editor. Difficult problems in hand surgery. St Louis (MO): Mosby; 1982. p. 169–72.

[25] Cooney WP, Lucca M, Chao E, et al. The kinesiology of the thumb trapeziometacarpal joint. J Bone Joint Surg 1981;63:1371–81.

[26] Cooney WP, Chao EY. Biomechanical analysis of static forces in the thumb during hand function. J Bone Joint Surg [Am] 1977;59:27–36.

[27] Imaeda T, An KN, Cooney WP. Functional anatomy and biomechanics of the thumb. Hand Clin 1992;8:9–15.

[28] Basmajian JV. The unsung virtue of ligaments. Surg Clin North Am 1974;54:1259–67.

[29] Cooney WP, An KN, Daube JR, et al. Electromyographic analysis of the thumb: a study of isometric forces in pinch and grasp. J Hand Surg [Am] 1985;10:202–10.

[30] Katarincic JA. Thumb kinematics and their relevance to function. Hand Clin 2001;17:169–74.

[31] von Oudenaarde E. Structure and function of the abductor pollicis longus muscle. J Anat 1991;174:221–7.

[32] Gonzalez MH, Sohlberg R, Brown A, et al. The first dorsal compartment: an anatomic study. J Hand Surg [Am] 1995;20:657–60.

[33] Brunelli GA, Brunelli GR. Anatomy of the extensor pollicis brevis muscle. J Hand Surg [Br] 1992;17:267–9.

[34] Linburg RM, Comstock BE. Anomalous tendon slips from the flexor pollicis longus to the flexor digitorum profundus. J Hand Surg [Am] 1979;4:79–83.

[35] Eyler DL, Markee JE. The anatomy and function of the intrinsic musculature of the fingers. J Bone Joint Surg [Am] 1954;36:1–9.

[36] Smith RJ. Intrinsic muscles of the fingers: function, dysfunction, and surgical reconstruction. In: AAOS Instructional Course Lecture; 1975. p. 200–20.

[37] von Schroeder HP, Botte MJ. The dorsal aponeurosis, intrinsic, hypothenar, and thenar musculature of the hand. Clin Orthop Relat Res 2001;383:97–107.

[38] Pellegrini VD Jr, Ku CW, Smith RL. Pathobiology of articular cartilage in trapeziometacarpal osteoarthritis. II. Surface ultrastructure by scanning electron microscopy. J Hand Surg [Am] 1994;19:79–85.

[39] Tomaino MM, King J, Leit M. Thumb basal joint arthritis. In: Green DP, Hotchkiss RN, Pederson WC, et al, editors. Green's operative hand surgery. 5th edition. Philadelphia: Elsevier; 2005. p. 461–85.

[40] Eaton R, Lane L, Littler JW, et al. Ligament reconstruction for the painful thumb carpometacarpal joint. A long term assessment. J Hand Surg [Am] 1984;9:692–9.

[41] Eaton R, Littler JW. Ligament reconstruction for the painful thumb carpometacarpal joint. J Bone Joint Surg Am 1973;55:1655–66.

[42] Eaton R, Littler JW. A study of the basal joint of the thumb. Treatment of its disabilities by fusion. J Bone Joint Surg Am 1969;51:661–8.

[43] Pellegrini VD Jr, Smith RL, Ku CW. Pathobiology of articular cartilage in trapeziometacarpal osteoarthritis. I. Regional biochemical analysis. J Hand Surg [Am] 1994;19:70–8.

[44] Pellegrini VD Jr, Olcott C, Hollenberg G, et al. Contact patterns in the trapeziometacarpal joint: effects of volar beak ligament division and extension metacarpal osteotomy. J Hand Surg [Am] 1993;18:238–44.

[45] Xu L, Strauch RJ, Ateshian GA, et al. Topography of the osteoarthritic thumb carpometacarpal joint and its variation with regard to gender, age, site, and osteoarthritic stage. J Hand Surg [Am] 1998;23:454–64.

[46] Ateshian GA, Ark JW, Rosenwasser MP, et al. Contact areas in the thumb carpometacarpal joint. J Orthop Res 1995;13:450–8.

[47] Pellegrini VD Jr. Fractures at the base of the thumb. Hand Clin 1988;4:87–102.

[48] Cullen JP, Parentis MA, Chinchilli VM, et al. Simulated Bennett fracture treated with closed reduction and percutaneous pinning: a biomechanical analysis of residual incongruity of the joint. J Bone Joint Surg 1997;79:420–3.

[49] Kirk JA, Ansell BM, Bywaters EG. The hypermobility syndrome: Musculoskeletal complaints associated with generalized joint hypermobility. Ann Rheum Dis 1967;26:419–25.

[50] Pellegrini VD Jr. Osteoarthritis at the base of the thumb. Orthop Clin North Am 1992;23:83–102.

[51] Molitor P, Emery R, Meggitt B. First metacarpal osteotomy for carpometacarpal osteoarthritis. J Hand Surg [Br] 1991;16:424–7.

[52] Wilson J. Basal osteotomy of the first metacarpal in the treatment of arthritis of the carpometacarpal joint of the thumb. Br J Surg 1973;60:854–8.

[53] Wilson J, Bossley C. Osteotomy in the treatment of osteoarthritis in the first carpometacarpal joint. J Bone Joint Surg Br 1983;65:179–81.

[54] Moulton MJ, Parentis MA, Kelly MJ, et al. Influence of metacarpophalangeal joint position on basal joint-loading in the thumb. J Bone Joint Surg Am 2001;83:709–16.

ELSEVIER
SAUNDERS

Hand Clin 24 (2008) 231–237

Physical Diagnosis and Radiographic Examination of the Thumb

Peter Tsai, MD, Pedro K. Beredjiklian, MD

Department of Orthopaedic Surgery, University of Pennsylvania School of Medicine,
Presbyterian Hospital, 3900 Market Street, Philadelphia, PA 19104, USA

The first evolutionary evidence of the modern thumb was discovered in 1960 at Olduvai Gorge in Tanzania. *Homo habilis* (handy man) had fingers resembling ape fingers, with their capacity for powerful flexion, but thumbs with features similar to those of the modern human thumb and its capacity for opposition. The interphalangeal joint (IPJ) and the metacarpophalangeal joint (MPJ) of the modern human provide the ability to flex and extend the thumb. The carpometacarpal joint (CMCJ) allows opposition to the fingers while providing a stable structure to protect the cartilagenous surfaces from excessive wear. To prevent dorsoradial migration of the metacarpal on the trapezium, chimpanzees have developed a long volar metacarpal beak, which engages the trapezium, limiting translation and rotation of the metacarpal on the trapezium [1]. In the evolutionary process, the human thumb has lost that bony beak and developed a corresponding ligament complex (thus the Darwinian term "volar beak" ligament) that allows stabilization of the CMCJ with lateral pinch [2].

The movement of the thumb as described by Kuczynski [3] involves rotation and translation between the trapezial ridge and the corresponding groove in the base of the thumb metacarpal. Motion across the CMCJ, MPJ, and IPJ are coordinated with thumb flexion and, in opposition, there is an obligate flexion and pronation of the thumb [4]. The CMCJ allows flexion/extension in the convex direction and abduction/adduction in the concave direction of the trapezium, with rotation occurring oblique to these axes [3].

There are 16 ligaments described by Bettinger [5] about the CMCJ, 7 of which are direct stabilizers of the joint. The ligaments understood to be most important for static and dynamic stability include the dorsoradial ligament and the deep anterior oblique ligament (volar beak ligament). There are different opinions regarding the importance of each of these ligaments. From an evolutionary standpoint, logic says the deep anterior oblique ligament is the most important for stability. However, biomechanical studies suggest that the dorsoradial ligament may be the primary static stabilizer of this joint [6].

The MPJ and IPJ allow flexion and extension in variable degrees of both with small amounts of radial and ulnar deviation as well as pronation and supination. Yoshida and associates [7], in a study evaluating volunteers and cadavers, found a flexion range between 40° and 126° with a mean of 77° and a range of extension from 0° to 72° with a mean of 35° extension in volunteer subjects. A prior study evaluating the effects of range of motion and injury prevalence showed a correlation between stiff thumbs and injury. The investigators hypothesized that stiff thumbs are less able to disperse forces than more mobile thumbs, thereby predisposing them to injury [8].

Prevalence

The thumb CMCJ has a high prevalence of osteoarthritis, typically in the older postmenopausal female population [9]. The reason the female thumb has a much higher predisposition for the development of osteoarthritis is unknown. Some investigators have argued that anatomic differences between genders may provide an explanation for this finding. Differences in the female CMCJ include (1) greater reciprocal curvature of the trapezium and metacarpal articular surfaces,

doi:10.1016/j.hcl.2008.03.004

hand.theclinics.com

(2) lower degree of congruity between the joint surfaces, and (3) smaller surface areas leading to increased contact stresses [1].

Several epidemiologic studies have attempted to quantify the incidence of CMCJ degenerative disease. The prevalence of the disease was found to be approximately 15% in a large Finnish study of adults over 30 years of age [10]. The prevalence of hand arthritis in females over 55 years of age approached 67% in another study, with 21% to 36% of the radiographic signs of arthritis occurring at the thumb CMCJ [11,12]. The Framingham study group in the United States showed the rate of CMCJ arthritis symptoms to be approximately 7% in females and 5% in males over the age of 70 years [13].

Other investigators have looked into the influence of genetic and environmental factors that may lead to the development of osteoarthritis. A recent study by Fontana and colleagues [14] delineate such risk factors for the development of CMCJ degenerative disease, including (1) occupations with repetitive thumb use and (2) family history. Another study of almost 4000 Finnish patients suggests strong correlation between obesity and thumb CMCJ arthritis [10]. Laxity at the thumb CMCJ has been long thought to be a predisposing factor, yet there has been only one longitudinal study to date examining the issue [15]. Hunter and colleagues examined radial subluxation on the Framingham study cohort and found a strong association between subluxation and thumb carpometacarpal arthritis. The investigators found that the more radially subluxated the metacarpal was, the higher the likelihood of developing arthritis of this joint.

In comparison to the interest devoted to research concerning the CMCJ, there is little data regarding the prevalence of degenerative disease of the thumb IPJ and MPJ. MPJ arthritis is common in those affected by systemic inflammatory arthritides, and in those with a history of a traumatic injury to the joint. For example, patients with chronic, untreated MPJ collateral ligament injuries leading to joint subluxation often present months or years later with signs and symptoms of joint degeneration.

Physical examination

Differential diagnosis

Patients who present with radial-sided hand and wrist pain must have a detailed physical examination of the hand and wrist. Pain on the radial side of the hand and wrist can be due to soft tissue and bony disorders. The differential diagnosis of radial-sided hand and wrist pain include (1) intersection syndrome (tendinopathy of the wrist extensors in the distal/radial forearm); (2) DeQuervain's tenosynovitis (tendinopathy of the tendons within the first dorsal compartment of the wrist); (3) injury (acute or chronic) of the scaphoid; (4) injury (acute or chronic) of the scapholunate interosseous ligament; (5) osteoarthritis of the scapho-trapezial-trapezoid (STT) joint; (6) instability, synovitis, or osteoarthritis of the CMCJ; (7) instability, synovitis, or osteoarthritis of the MPJ; (8) stenosing tenosynovitis of the thumb (trigger thumb); and (9) osteoarthritis of the IPJ of the thumb.

Inspection

The patient who presents with basal joint arthritis may complain of palmar-sided pain at the base of the metacarpal. On inspection, the patient may have the "shoulder sign," prominence at the base of the metacarpal with a step off between the thumb metacarpal and the more proximal trapezium, typically in a dorsoradial direction. This prominence may be due to inflammation, subluxation of the metacarpal on the trapezium, or osteophytes resulting from the degenerative process. In most cases, swelling about the joint is visible in patients with symptomatic degenerative disease. In a subset of patients, the thumb MPJ may be hyperextended. It has been theorized that this extension is compensatory in nature. Due to the degenerative changes, the base of the metacarpal can be stiff or contracted in adducted position. In an effort to extend the thumb, patients with baseline hypermobility of the MPJ will overextend the joint. In a challenge to this conventional wisdom, Moulton and colleagues [16] have posited that the MPJ extension may actually be a causative factor in the formation of arthritis at the CMCJ. With extension at the MPJ, there is reciprocal flexion of the metacarpal, which causes contact pressures to migrate dorsally on the trapezium, affecting the CMCJ mechanics and eventually initiating the cascade of events leading to osteoarthritis. In patients with weakness due to disuse or those with concomitant severe carpal tunnel syndrome, loss of bulk and atrophy of the thenar musculature of the hand can also be readily visible. Finally, in severe cases of osteoarthritis, an adduction contracture of the thumb metacarpal may also be observed.

Patients with complaints related to the MPJ and IPJ of the thumb present with swelling about the joints, due to either proliferation of the synovial lining of the joint or osteophytes. In patients where chronic injury of the MPJ collateral ligaments has led to degenerative changes, obvious deformity of the proximal phalanx (radially or volarly directed) can be readily determined. In addition, patients with osteoarthritis often have cystic masses, termed mucoid cysts, on the dorsal aspect of the IPJ. These mucoid cysts represent cystic lesions that communicate with the joint, and are often associated with a dorsal osteophyte. Larger cysts about the IPJ located about the germinal matrix create grooving and deformity of the nail plate. Patients affected with inflammatory arthropathies can show skin or nail deformities related to their systemic process, such as rheumatoid nodules in patients with rheumatoid arthritis or nail pitting in patients with psoriatic arthritis.

Palpation

Patients affected with arthritic changes in the joints of the thumb classically complain of pain in the region of the affected joint on application of manual pressure. Patients affected with CMCJ arthritis have pain on palpation over the joint that can be localized to the volar side directly below the thenar eminence of the thumb (Fig. 1). In the early stages of disease, instability of the CMCJ can be detected by stabilizing the trapezium and manipulating the thumb metacarpal in a dorsal/volar direction. In addition, the carpometacarpal

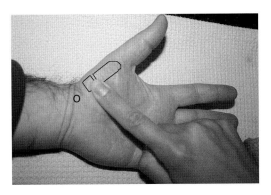

Fig. 1. Palpation of the volar aspect of the thumb CMCJ elicits pain in patients with joint degeneration. The distal pole of the scaphoid is marked with a circle, and the metacarpal and trapezium are outlined.

"grind test" elicits discomfort when an axially directed force is applied on the thumb metacarpal. This provocative maneuver increases the contact stresses on the CMCJ, leading to pain and often a palpable crepitance on manipulation of the joint. Patients with changes over the MPJ and IPJ also have tenderness on palpation. Similar to the CMCJ, patients with early changes due to chronic collateral ligament disruption may display MPJ instability. This instability can be detected by placing the MPJ in flexion and applying a radially or ulnarly directed stress on the proximal phalanx. In patients affected with inflammatory arthritides, the MPJ can assume a flexed position due to subluxation of the extensor pollicis longus tendon with resultant IPJ extension due to the increased forces acting at the IPJ. If the MPJ has assumed an extended position due to synovial proliferation and attrition of the stabilizing structures, the IPJ will assume a flexed position due to increased pull from the flexor pollicis longus tendon. These reciprocal deformities are compensatory and largely seen in patients with systemic inflammatory changes.

Strength and range of motion

Assessment of strength and range of motion is also important. Strength is often limited in patients with CMCJ degenerative changes, and is primarily affected in pinch strength testing. Using commercially available devices, the determination of key and tip pinch strength is readily made, and should be compared with that of the contralateral side. Range of motion is almost always limited, and correlates with the degree of degenerative changes in the joint. The determination of CMCJ range of motion can be difficult. Typical range of motion for the normal CMCJ is $53°$ ($\pm11°$) of flexion and extension, and $42°$ ($\pm4°$) of abduction and adduction. Range of motion of the MPJ and IPJ is highly variable between individuals, and a comparison with the contralateral side is important.

Provocative maneuvers

Provocative maneuvers for CMCJ arthritis and other conditions affecting the radial hand/wrist are listed in Table 1.

A careful neurologic examination should also be performed as part of the complete physical evaluation. An association between carpal tunnel syndrome and CMCJ arthritis has been established in one study, where 43% of patients

Table 1
Differential diagnosis and physical examination of CMCJ arthritis

Diagnosis	Physical examination
Intersection syndrome	Pain and crepitation with wrist flexion and extension over the intersection between the first and second extensor compartments in the radial forearm
DeQuervain's tenosynovitis	Pain over the first dorsal compartment; positive Finkelstein's test (radial wrist pain with radial deviation of the wrist while the thumb is held in a flexed position)
Scaphoid injury (acute or chronic)	Pain over the anatomic snuffbox
Scapholunate interosseous ligament injury (acute or chronic)	Pain in the wrist distal to Lister's tubercle; positive scaphoid shift test
STT joint arthritis	Tenderness distal to the scaphoid
Stenosing tenosynovitis	Tenderness on the palmar aspect of the MPJ; locking in flexion of the IPJ

evaluated or treated for CMCJ degenerative changes also met the criteria for carpal tunnel syndrome [17].

Radiographic studies

Radiographic evaluation is critical for the evaluation and staging of patients with arthritis of the joints of the thumb, although the indications for treatment should be based primarily on the patient's complaints of pain, weakness, and functional disability. The radiographic assessment of these joints primarily and most commonly includes plain radiographs, although other modalities, such as technetium bone scanning or MRI, can be helpful (Fig. 2).

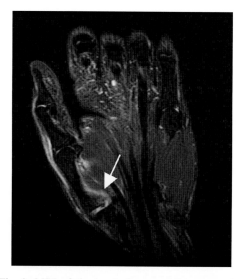

Fig. 2. MRI of the hand. A coronal fat suppression image of the thumb CMCJ displaying increased signal intensity about the area of the volar beak ligament (*white arrow*) in a patient with a history of joint instability.

Plain radiographs

Plain radiographs show changes typical of either degenerative or inflammatory joint degeneration. In cases of degenerative (primary or post-traumatic osteoarthritis), radiographic changes reveal asymmetric joint narrowing, sclerosis, subluxation, and osteophyte formation. In those affected with inflammatory arthritis, radiographs reveal symmetric joint narrowing, periarticular osteopenia, periarticular erosions, subluxation, and, in some cases, significant disruption of the joint architecture.

The plain radiographic evaluation of the IPJ and MPJ of the thumb typically involves assessment in the posteroanterior, lateral, and oblique views. Plain radiograph evaluation of the thumb CMCJ includes a true anteroposterior view as described by Roberts, taken by placing the forearm in maximum pronation with the dorsal aspect of the thumb resting on the x-ray table (Fig. 3). In addition, a true lateral view of the CMCJ can be obtained by pronating the hand about 20° degrees, placing the thumb flat on the x-ray table, and angling the x-ray beam about 10° from vertical in the distal to proximal projection. Finally, stress views may also be helpful to determine the amount of dynamic instability of the joint.

In 1973, Eaton and Littler devised a radiographic staging scheme that correlates with progression of arthritic changes in the CMCJ. The scheme has since been modified [18,19]:

Stage 1: Articular contours normal; joint space may be widened due to synovitis. There should be less than one-third subluxation of the articular surfaces on any view (see Fig. 3).

Stage 2: Slight narrowing of the joint space with osteophytes measuring less than 2 mm

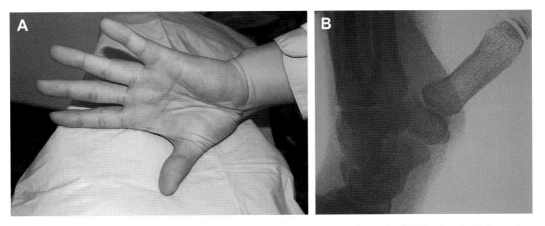

Fig. 3. (*A*) Clinical photograph demonstrating the position of the hand to evaluate the CMCJ using the Roberts view. (*B*) Radiograph of the Roberts view with Eaton stage 1 CMCJ disease.

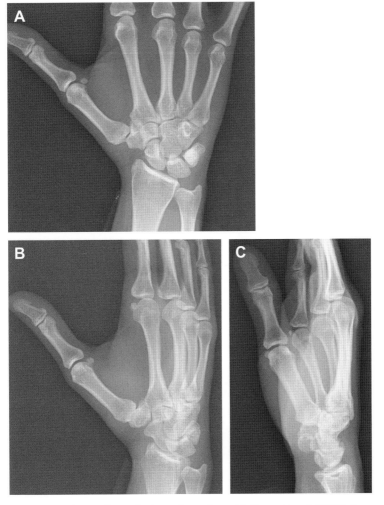

Fig. 4. (*A–C*) Three radiograph views of a patient with Eaton stage 2 CMCJ disease.

in size. The articular contours remain normal, and there may more than one-third subluxation of the joint surfaces apparent on stress radiographs (Fig. 4).

Stage 3: CMCJ narrowing with sclerotic or cystic changes in subchondral bone and osteophytes measuring more than 2 mm in size. The STT joint remains intact (Fig. 5).

Stage 4: Pantrapezial arthrosis. Both the CMCJ and STT joint are affected with severe articular degeneration.

Though widely used, the reliability of this classification scheme has been questioned, with one study revealing the intrarater reliability to be 66%, while the interrater reliability was 60% amongst a group of three hand surgeons [20]. One Danish epidemiologic study showed a statistical correlation between subchondral sclerosis and clinically significant self-reported pain [21]. The trapezial tilt angle is another parameter that can be used to determine the severity of basal joint disease. It is defined as the complement angle between the longitudinal axis of the second metacarpal and a line tangent to the middle of the trapezial articular surface on the Robert view and was found to correlate with the Eaton staging [22].

The presence of STT arthritis on plain radiographs can be difficult to establish. In a cadaveric study, Brown and colleagues [23] examined the correlation between radiographic and visualized arthritic changes at the STT joint at the time of

surgery, and found a correlation between radiographic and grossly visible changes of the joint in only 39% of cases. These findings contrast with those described by North and Eaton [24] in 1983. In that study, the investigators concluded that radiographs overestimated the extent of disease at the STT joint. This study showed 73% of STT joints had radiograph changes on evaluation before surgery for the CMCJ, but intraoperatively only 46% were noted on direct inspection to be affected by arthritis [24].

Other imaging

MRI can be used for the detection of suspected soft tissue injuries, particularly the stabilizing ligamentous structures. MRI can demonstrate synovial proliferation within the joints and degeneration of articular cartilage, which may not be obvious on plain radiographs. It will reveal synovitis, loss of articular hyaline cartilage (best seen in the T2-weighted images), and evidence of chronic soft tissue disruption in those patients with chronic ligamentous injuries. MRI can also be of help in determining the presence or absence of other conditions in the differential diagnosis of thumb pain.

Technetium bone scanning, while not a very specific diagnostic test, is highly sensitive for the detection of pathology in bony and soft tissue structures about the thumb. It is of most help in selected cases where the diffuse nature of symptoms clouds the clinical assessment of a given patient, helping to objectively establish a specific area of pathology. In the few cases in which bone scanning is used as a diagnostic modality for the assessment of arthritic changes, concentrated radiotracer uptake is seen in the periarticular structures. Finally, it is helpful in establishing the diagnosis of complex regional pain syndrome type I in patients with diffuse thumb and wrist pain after injury or surgery with dystrophic skin changes on physical examination.

Summary

Arthritis of the thumb joints is a common problem and remains a significant cause of morbidity in the adult population. Careful physical examination is critical in the assessment of these patients, given the large differential diagnosis of conditions affecting the thumb and the radial side of the wrist. Because treatment should be specifically directed at the area of pathology,

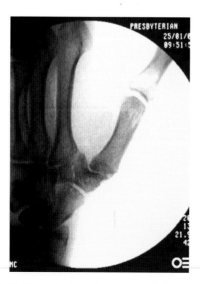

Fig. 5. Radiograph view of a patient with Eaton stage 3 CMCJ disease.

adequate diagnosis is vital. Plain radiograph evaluation remains the diagnostic modality of choice in the evaluation of patients with degenerative conditions about the hand and wrist.

References

[1] Marzke MW, Marzke RF. Evolution of the human hand: approaches to acquiring, analysing and interpreting the anatomical evidence. J Anat 2000; 197(1):121–40.

[2] Marzke MW. Evolutionary development of the human thumb. Hand Clin 1992;8(1):1–8.

[3] Kuczynski K. Carpometacarpal joint of the human thumb. J Anat 1974;118(1):119–26.

[4] Li ZM, Tang J. Coordination of thumb joints during opposition. J Biomech 2007;40(3):502–10.

[5] Bettinger PC, Berger RA. Functional ligamentous anatomy of the trapezium and trapeziometacarpal joint (gross and arthroscopic). Hand Clin 2001; 17(2):151–68.

[6] Colman M, Mass DP, Draganich LF. Effects of the deep anterior oblique and dorsoradial ligaments on trapeziometacarpal joint stability. J Hand Surg [Am] 2007;32(3):310–7.

[7] Yoshida R, House HO, Patterson RM, et al. Motion and morphology of the thumb metacarpophalangeal joint. J Hand Surg [Am] 2003;28(5):753–7.

[8] Shaw SJ, Morris MA. The range of motion of the metacarpo-phalangeal joint of the thumb and its relationship to injury. J Hand Surg [Br] 1992;17(2): 164–6.

[9] Pellegrini VD. The ABJS 2005 Nicolas Andry Award: osteoarthritis and injury at the base of the human thumb: survival of the fittest? Clin Orthop Relat Res 2005;438:266–76.

[10] Haara MM, Heliövaara M, Kröger H, et al. Osteoarthritis in the carpometacarpal joint of the thumb. Prevalence and associations with disability and mortality. J Bone Joint Surg Am 2004;86-A(7):1452–7.

[11] Dahaghin S, Bierma-Zeinstra SM, Ginai AZ, et al. Prevalence and pattern of radiographic hand osteoarthritis and association with pain and disability (the Rotterdam study). Ann Rheum Dis 2005;64(5): 682–7.

[12] Wilder FV, Barrett JP, Farina EJ. Joint-specific prevalence of osteoarthritis of the hand. Osteoarthritis Cartilage 2006;14(9):953–7.

[13] Zhang Y, Niu J, Kelly-Hayes M, et al. Prevalence of symptomatic hand osteoarthritis and its impact on functional status among the elderly: The Framingham Study. Am J Epidemiol 2002;156(11): 1021–7.

[14] Fontana L, Neel S, Claise JM, et al. Osteoarthritis of the thumb carpometacarpal joint in women and occupational risk factors: a case-control study. J Hand Surg [Am] 2007;32(4):459–65.

[15] Hunter DJ, Zhang Y, Sokolove J, et al. Trapeziometacarpal subluxation predisposes to incident trapeziometacarpal osteoarthritis (OA): the Framingham Study. Osteoarthritis Cartilage 2005;13(11):953–7.

[16] Moulton MJ, Parentis MA, Kelly MJ, et al. Influence of metacarpophalangeal joint position on basal joint-loading in the thumb. J Bone Joint Surg 2001; 83-A(5):709–16.

[17] Florack TM, Miller RJ, Pellegrini VD, et al. The prevalence of carpal tunnel syndrome in patients with basal joint arthritis of the thumb. J Hand Surg [Am] 1992;17(4):624–30.

[18] Eaton RG, Littler JW. Ligament reconstruction for the painful thumb carpometacarpal joint. J Bone Joint Surg 1973;55-A(8):1655–66.

[19] Cooke KS, Singson RD, Glickel SZ, et al. Degenerative changes of the trapeziometacarpal joint: radiologic assessment. Skeletal Radiol 1995;24(7): 523–7.

[20] Kubik NJ, Lubahn JD. Intrarater and interrater reliability of the Eaton classification of basal joint arthritis. J Hand Surg [Am] 2002;27(5):882–5.

[21] Sonne-Holm S, Jacobsen S. Osteoarthritis of the first carpometacarpal joint: a study of radiology and clinical epidemiology. Results from the Copenhagen Osteoarthritis Study. Osteoarthritis Cartilage 2006; 14(5):496–500.

[22] Bettinger PC, Linscheid RL, Cooney WP 3rd, et al. Trapezial tilt: a radiographic correlation with advanced trapeziometacarpal joint arthritis. J Hand Surg [Am] 2001;26(4):692–7.

[23] Brown GD, Roh MS, Srauch RJ, et al. Radiography and visual pathology of the osteoarthritic scaphotrapezio-trapezoidal joint, and its relationship to trapeziometacarpal osteoarthritis. J Hand Surg [Am] 2003;28(5):739–43.

[24] North ER, Eaton RG. Degenerative joint disease of the trapezium: a comparative radiographic and anatomic study. J Hand Surg [Am] 1983;8(2): 160–6.

ELSEVIER
SAUNDERS

Hand Clin 24 (2008) 239–250

HAND
CLINICS

Treatment of Thumb Metacarpophalangeal and Interphalangeal Joint Arthritis

Eon K. Shin, MD[a],*, A. Lee Osterman, MD[b]

[a]Thomas Jefferson University Hospital, The Philadelphia Hand Center, P.C., 834 Chestnut Street, Suite G114, Philadelphia, PA 19107, USA
[b]Thomas Jefferson University Hospital, The Philadelphia Hand Center, P.C., 700 South Henderson Road, Suite 200, King of Prussia, PA 19406, USA

Osteoarthritis is a common disease of the articular cartilage. In patients older than 75, more than 80% have symptoms of osteoarthritis, making it one of the most expensive and debilitating diseases in terms of cost of diagnosis and therapy, complications of therapy, and lost productivity [1]. The arthritic process leads to erosion of articular cartilage, development of bone spurs, and progressive joint deformity. Subchrondral cysts commonly are seen on radiographs. Patients may present with subsequent loss of motion, instability, and chronic pain.

The presentation of thumb metacarpophalangeal (MCP) and interphalangeal (IP) osteoarthritis is not often described in the hand surgery literature. Although the exact incidence of thumb MCP and IP degenerative joint disease is ill defined, it is seen less commonly in a typical hand surgeon's practice than carpometacarpal (CMC) arthritis at the thumb base. Many of the surgical techniques developed for treatment of thumb arthritic conditions were designed with rheumatoid patients in mind.

The purpose of this review is to discuss the epidemiology of thumb MCP and IP degenerative joint disease, conservative therapies that may be undertaken before surgical intervention, and operative techniques that should be a part of every hand surgeon's armamentarium.

Etiology

Osteoarthritis

Primary thumb osteoarthritis typically presents at the CMC articulation. Epidemiologic studies have demonstrated a gender differential with women affected six times more frequently than men [2]. This difference may be the result of anatomic variations between the sexes [3,4]. There also is evidence to suggest that CMC osteoarthritis is related to repetitive activities, particularly in women [5].

Osteoarthritis affecting the thumb MCP and IP joints is far less common. To the authors' knowledge, surprisingly little information is available regarding the prevalence of primary osteoarthritis occurring more distally in the thumb. Previous reports have suggested that chronic repetitive trauma in patients who have heavy labor occupations may contribute to the development of osteoarthritis [6]. The index and middle finger MCP joints, however, typically are implicated in these cases.

Mechanical stress is postulated as playing an important role in the development of thumb IP joint osteoarthritis. Hunter and colleagues [7] conducted a population-based survey of elderly Chinese individuals living in Beijing to determine if there was any association between thumb IP degenerative joint disease and chopstick use. Chopsticks, used universally as eating utensils in China, increase joint loading in the first through third digits. This epidemiologic study found radiographic evidence of thumb IP joint osteoarthritis in 26% of the 2507 elderly individuals queried.

* Corresponding author.
E-mail address: ekshin@handcenters.com (E.K. Shin).

0749-0712/08/$ - see front matter. Published by Elsevier Inc.
doi:10.1016/j.hcl.2008.03.007

hand.theclinics.com

Statistical analysis demonstrated that chopstick use accounted for 19% of the risk for osteoarthritis developing in this joint in men and 36% of the risk in women.

Handedness is not shown to have a clear association with the development of thumb MCP and IP degenerative joint disease [8,9]. Lane and colleagues [8] compared dominant with nondominant hands of 134 consecutive community subjects ages 53 to 75 by questionnaire, radiographs of hands, and rheumatologic evaluation. These subjects estimated dominant hand use to be 2 to 10 times the amount of the nondominant hand. Although osteoarthritis was found in 133 of 134 subjects, no radiologic or clinical differences were found between the dominant and nondominant hands. Further investigation into the causes of primary osteoarthritis of the thumb is warranted.

Secondary arthritis of the thumb MCP joint is more common after injuries that damage the ligaments on the ulnar or radial side of the MCP joint and that result in lateral instability of the joint [6]. Secondary MCP arthritis may result from thumb CMC joint disease and must be attended to at the time CMC joint reconstruction is performed. Other causes of osteoarthritis affecting the MCP and IP articulations include trauma, infection, and congenital abnormality. These conditions can expose the affected joint to a flood of cartilage and bone debris. Phagocytic cells in the synovial membrane then work to remove the debris from the synovial fluid, inciting a cycle of chronic inflammatory changes within the joint space.

Gout

Gout represents a disorder of nucleic acid metabolism leading to hyperuricemia and hyperuricosuria with ensuing monosodium urate crystal deposition in joints. These crystals activate inflammatory mediators, such as proteases, chemotactic factors, prostaglandins, leukotriene B4, and free oxygen radicals, which can cause intense swelling, erythema, and pain. Recurrent gouty arthritic attacks are characteristic, particularly in men between 40 and 60 years of age. Crystal deposition in the subcutaneous tissues, known as tophi, and renal stones also are commonly observed. A longitudinal study of 1337 healthy medical students demonstrated a cumulative lifetime incidence of 8% and identified significant risk factors, such as obesity, hypertension, and weight gain at an early age [10].

The diagnosis of gout can be made only by joint aspiration and inspection for crystals. A high level of suspicion should be maintained as gout often is called "the great imitator" and can mimic septic arthritis, rheumatoid arthritis, or neoplasm. Radiographic findings include soft tissue densities (tophi), intra-articular erosions at the joint margins, and extra-articular erosions. Gout typically affects the metatarsophalangeal joint of the first toe in 75% of patients, a condition called podagra. It also is observed commonly at the thumb MCP joint. Gout can affect the knees, ankles, elbows, wrists, and other finger joints.

Preoperative planning

A complete evaluation of patients presenting with thumb MCP or IP arthritis includes a thorough history and physical examination. The skin should be examined for possible mucous cyst formation, particularly about the IP joint or proximal to the thumbnail. Pain levels should be assessed carefully. Difficulties with activities of daily living also should be discussed. Static and dynamic deformities should be observed carefully (Fig. 1). The arcs of motion should be measured before treatment. Normal thumb MCP motion is between 0° and 56°, whereas normal IP joint motion is between −5° and 73° [11]. A functional arc of motion between 10° and 32° (mean 21°) for thumb MCP joints and between 2° and 43° (mean 18°) for IP joints is considered necessary for most activities of daily living [11]. If the upper extremity is used for ambulatory assistive devices, such as a cane or walker,

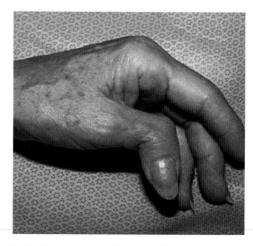

Fig. 1. Static angular deformity of the thumb interphalangeal joint.

then the durability of any proposed surgical recon-struction becomes more significant.

Imaging studies of the affected sites should be obtained. Standard anteroposterior and lateral radiographs give sufficient information about the thumb MCP and IP joints to make determinations about joint preservation versus salvage procedures (Fig. 2). CT or MRI scans rarely are indicated.

Nonoperative treatment

Conservative therapies for patients who have osteoarthritis and rheumatoid arthritis are similar. Pain medicines, such as nonsteroidal anti-inflam-matory drugs (NSAIDs), should be attempted first. Despite the many NSAIDs available, no single compound has been found more efficacious than another [12]. In addition, chronic use of NSAIDs or oral corticosteroids for isolated thumb joint arthritis is not recommended as the long-term side effects far outweigh the potential benefits. Gastric mucosal ulcers have been visual-ized endoscopically in 20% of patients using NSAIDs for 6 months and 1% to 2% of these patients develop hemorrhage or perforation. For-tunately, 90% of these lesions heal after discontin-uation of the NSAID and use of acid-reducing medication [13–15].

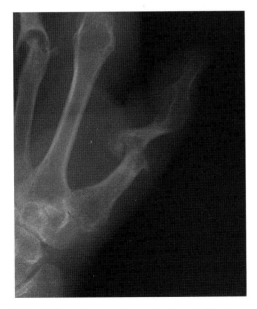

Fig. 2. Plain radiograph demonstrating significant ero-sive osteoarthritis affecting the metacarpophalangeal articulation.

For patients who have gout, appropriate medical therapies should be instituted to prevent symptomatic flares. Initial treatment generally is with indomethicin or colchicine. Allopurinol is used to lower serum uric acid levels in hyper-uricemic patients who have chronic gout and is given before chemotherapy for patients who have myeloproliferative disorders.

Activity modifications and splint immobiliza-tion also may be beneficial to prevent capsular inflammation or synovitis. For immobilization of the thumb MCP and IP joints, typically a hand-based thumb spica splint is sufficient and allows most activities of daily living. A brief course of immobilization for 4 to 6 weeks may be sufficient to resolve thumb pain secondary to synovitis.

Corticosteroid injections are helpful in pa-tients who have mild joint involvement, particu-larly at the MCP articulation. Injection solutions typically consist of a 50:50 mixture of 1% lidocaine without epinephrine and methylpred-nisolone or triamcinolone. To the authors' knowledge, no clinical studies have been per-formed comparing various corticosteroid formu-lations for safety and efficacy. Few complications from intra-articular corticosteroid injections are reported, however, suggesting that low intermit-tent doses pose little risk for significant adverse effects [16]. There is controversy as to whether or not corticosteroid injections have a protective or deleterious effect on the remaining cartilage [17]. Reported complications include corticosteroid ar-thropathy, tendon rupture, postinjection flare, and hypersensitivity reactions. Patients should be advised that a transient increase in discomfort can occur for several days after injection and that the medication does not take effect until 3 to 7 days later.

Surgical techniques

Patients suffering from thumb pain secondary to arthritis may require surgery when medical management has failed to relieve the pain or when digit deformity is interfering with hand function and activities of daily living. Surgical procedures can improve function and relieve pain greatly, allowing patients to maintain independence and improve their quality of life. Various surgical options include arthroscopic synovectomy, ar-throplasty, and arthrodesis for the MCP joint. Few options are available for treatment of the thumb IP joint.

Thumb metacarpophalangeal joint

Arthroscopy

In patients who have mild osteoarthritis or synovitis of the MCP joint, arthroscopic synovectomy permits a diagnostic and therapeutic approach. Open synovectomies are difficult because of poor visualization and limited access to all regions of the joint and can lead to considerable stiffness after surgery. Although thumb arthroscopy has gained considerable popularity for treatment of CMC pathology [18,19], the technique is not used commonly at the MCP level.

For visualization of the MCP joint, a 30° arthroscope that is 1.9 mm in diameter is necessary. A 2.0-mm shaver usually is the main operative instrument although small radiofrequency probes also are used. Once appropriate anesthesia is administered, a patient's hand is suspended with a single Chinese fingertrap on the thumb. Approximately 5 to 10 pounds of traction is adequate. The appropriate level for arthroscope entry is determined by insufflating the joint with sterile saline and inserting a small curved clamp into the joint space. The arthroscope then can be introduced at the same angle in an atraumatic fashion. The portals lie on either side of the extensor mechanism. The second portal can be created under direct visualization.

To visualize the capsule and ligamentous structures, a complete synovectomy must be performed intially to permit full inspection of the MCP joint. A radiofrequency probe also can be used for this purpose. The articular surface of the metacarpal head and proximal phalanx then is assessed. An arthroscopic evaluation helps to determine the location and extent of injury and also gives an opportunity to render treatment by simple débridement or by thermal capsulorraphy. The arthroscope then is removed and the portals closed with Steri-Strips.

Arthroplasty

If an MCP joint demonstrates extensive degenerative changes as seen arthroscopically or if patient radiographs demonstrate significant joint disease refractory to conservative care, MCP arthroplasty is an option for patients who desire motion-preserving measures. In rheumatoid patients, Swanson silicone implants have been popularized for use in finger MCP joints. The shortcomings of silicone implants, however, include implant fracture, bone reaction adjacent to the implant, implant dislocation, and silicone synovitis. Silicone implants rarely are used for patients who have primary or secondary osteoarthritis given the greater functional demands of this patient population.

In 1973, Steffee [20] introduced a two-part polyethylene and metal thumb MCP arthroplasty system (Fig. 3). Although typically used in rheumatoid patients, its use also is described in patients who have posttraumatic osteoarthritis [21]. A dorsal longitudinal incision between the extensor pollicis brevis and the extensor pollicis longus tendons is made directly over the MCP joint. The collateral ligaments are incised and the joint is hyperflexed to expose the cartilaginous surfaces. Once the joint surfaces are excised perpendicular to the longitudinal axes of the metacarpal and proximal phalanx, the intramedullary canals are prepared using a curette or side cutting burr. After the canals are cleaned, polymethylmethacrylate cement is introduced under pressure into the canals. The components then are seated, ensuring that the prosthesis is oriented properly. The components are snap-locked together and the motion evaluated. The wound then is closed in layers. The

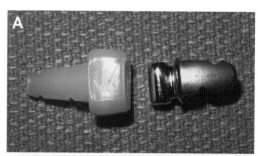

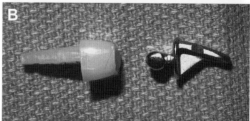

Fig. 3. The Steffee metacarpophalangeal joint implant is a two-part polyethylene and metal hinged prosthesis. The distal metal component is snap-locked into the proximal polyethylene portion and allows for hinged flexion and extension movement. (*A*) Dorsal and (*B*) lateral views of the components. (*From* McGovern RM, Shin AY, Beckenbaugh RD, et al. Long-term results of cemented Stefee arthroplasty of the thumb metacarpophalangeal joint. J Hand Surg [Am] 2001;26:115–22; with permission.)

MCP joint is held in extension with a thumb spica splint.

Recently, pyrolytic carbon (pyrocarbon) implants (Ascension Orthopedics, Austin, Texas) have gained increasing popularity for treatment of finger MCP and IP degenerative joint disease. Their use in the thumb has been limited to date. Nevertheless, pyrocarbon implants show promise for strength, durability, and biologic inertia. The elastic modulus of pyrocarbon is similar to that of cortical bone with excellent fatigue and wear characteristics. It is best reserved for patients in whom soft tissues and collateral ligaments are preserved.

The approach to the MCP joint is through a dorsal longitudinal or curvilinear incision. A starter awl is used to puncture the metacarpal head just volar to the dorsal surface of the metacarpal head. Under fluoroscopic visualization, the awl should be aligned with the long axis of the metacarpal's medullary canal. A metacarpal osteotomy then is made with a cutting guide, which provides 27.5° of distal tilt from the vertical.

A starter awl is used to puncture the base of the proximal phalanx. The position of the awl again is confirmed under fluoroscopy. A phalangeal base osteotomy is made tilted 5° distally from vertical. Initially, a conservative osteotomy should be made to allow for joint space adjustment later during the fitting of the trial implants. The collateral ligaments should be carefully preserved to provide for joint stability once the final implants are placed. The medullary canals of the metacarpal and proximal phalanx are broached, starting with the smallest size. The size of the phalangeal medullary canal generally is the limiting factor in implant size determination. The trial implants are placed and the joint reduced to assess stability, joint laxity, and range of motion. The final components then are impacted into place. A bulky splint is applied, maintaining the MCP joint in full extension. A carefully supervised program of therapy is initiated approximately 1 week after surgery.

Arthrodesis

Arthrodesis is an excellent and effective treatment of MCP joint pathology in the arthritic thumb. An important function of the MCP joint is stability; motion easily can be sacrificed to reduce pain and deformity and to achieve a stable thumb skeleton. The many techniques used for arthrodesis of the small finger joints also are applicable to the thumb. These include Kirschner wire fixation [22], tension band wiring techniques, bone screws, association osteosyntheses (AO) screws using the lag screw technique [23], bone pegs, and plate fixation.

The MCP joint has larger bones and bone surfaces than the IP joint. Therefore, acceptance of screw fixation is not an issue. To have good bone purchase at the head of the screw proximally and the screw threads distally, however, relatively larger screws must be used in an oblique or intramedullary fashion. Therefore, the bony resection and removal that may be required can be significant. Moreover, to use an AO lag screw, surgeons may be forced to remove a significant amount of cortical bone from the dorsal surface of the metacarpal to allow adequate seating of the screw head in an antegrade position. Therefore, Kirschner wires supplemented by tension bands provide an excellent surgical alternative (Fig. 4). There usually is sufficient bone stock to allow for this technique, and minimal bone removal is required.

Bone can be fashioned through flat cuts or the cup-and-cone technique of Carroll and Hill [24]. Two longitudinal Kirschner wires, 0.035 inches or 0.045 inches, are passed antegrade from the distal metaphyseal portion of the metacarpal down the intramedullary space of the proximal phalanx to engage the palmar cortex at the midportion of the proximal phalanx. A transverse bone tunnel is made with a Kirschner wire in the junction of the proximal first third to the proximal first half of the proximal phalanx. A 25-gauge wire is passed through the bone tunnel, looped in a figure eight fashion over the longitudinal pins, and tightened. The extensor mechanism is repaired with 5–0 nonabsorbable suture, and the skin is closed. Temporary splinting is provided and, depending on the patient, early mobilization is possible with good bone stock and adequate surgical technique in compliant patients.

In general, the MCP joint of the thumb should be fixed in a position of mild flexion, approximately 15°, as recommended by Inglis and colleagues [25]. Additionally, there should be mild abduction of the proximal phalanx and internal rotation or pronation to allow the thumb to pinch against the digits. The most important consideration, however, is the position of the thumb relative to the opposing digits.

Thumb interphalangeal joint

Arthrodesis

At the IP joint, arthrodesis is the mainstay of treatment of significant pain or deformity secondary to joint disease. The approach can be

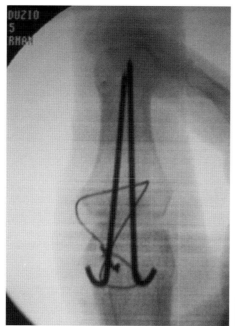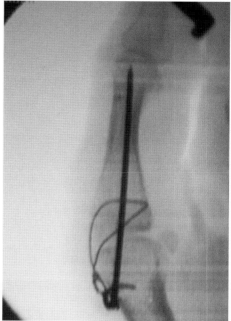

Fig. 4. Tension band construct for thumb metacarpophalangeal joint arthrodesis.

performed through a longitudinal incision, a dorsal zigzag, an S-shaped curve, an H-shaped incision, or a Y-shaped incision [26]. After exposure of the extensor mechanism through joint flexion and collateral ligament incision, it can be divided transversely to allow for joint access. Using a rongeur and curette, the articular cartilage is removed to expose subchondral bone. Bone contouring can be performed to accommodate the base of the distal phalanx to the head of the proximal phalanx, or converted to a cup-and-cone arrangement.

Methods of arthrodesis vary widely and include fixation with Kirschner wires, headless compression screws, and external devices [24]. Fixation with a headless screw provides the advantage of minimal splinting and early mobilization [27,28]. Various headless compression screw systems feature drilling of a guide wire antegrade down the medullary canal of the distal phalanx after preparation of the denuded joint space. The guide wire then is drilled retrograde back across the joint and into the medullary canal of the manually reduced proximal phalanx. The position of the wire is confirmed under fluoroscopic visualization. Self-tapping screws then are positioned over the guide wire and across the IP joint, taking care to bury the screw head fully within the tuft of the distal phalanx.

In the distal IP (DIP) joints of the fingers, care must be taken to ensure that the screw threads do not penetrate through the distal phalangeal cortex, which can lead to disruption of the nail bed and permanent nail deformity. In a cadaveric study, Wyrsch and colleagues [29] found penetration of the dorsal distal phalangeal cortex by screw threads in 83% of specimens and in all female specimens during joint instrumentation with a Herbert screw. This can result in loss of purchase by the screw and may require supplementation with an additional Kirschner wire. This usually is not problematic in the thumb given the larger size of the medullary canal. Sometimes the diameter of the metaphysis of the proximal phalanx is so large that the screw does not gain purchase. If preoperative radiographs suggest this, alternate means of fixation should be used (Fig. 5).

For osteoarthritis patients, Kirschner wire fixation may be the most expedient solution. Bone quality is not as significant an issue as it may be in rheumatoid patients. Generally, 0.045 inches is the minimum viable size for Kirschner wires. The IP joint ideally should be established in 15° to 25° of flexion. Two crossed Kirshner wires can be drilled longitudinally retrograde from the distal pulp across the IP joint into the proximal phalanx.

A novel technique of IP joint arthrodesis is featured by the X-Fuse system (Memometal, Memphis, Tennessee). The X-Fuse system allows intramedullary placement of an implant after IP

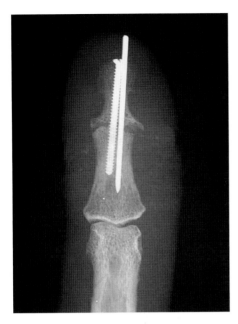

Fig. 5. Supplementary Kirschner wire fixation may be required for thumb interphalangeal joint arthrodesis, given the larger diameter of the medullary canals and the poor rotational control a single screw may provide.

joint preparation and permits predetermined amounts of flexion at the fusion site. Although specifically designed for DIP joint fusion in the fingers, the X-Fuse system will soon be modified for use at the thumb IP joint. The approach to the IP joint is identical to other methodologies. The proximal phalanx is prepared first using a small reamer and drill. Rasps of increasing size then are placed into the medullary canal of the proximal phalanx (Fig. 6A). The distal phalanx is prepared similarly (see Fig. 6B). Once positioning of the trial implant is confirmed under fluoroscopic visualization, the actual prosthesis is impacted into place (see Fig. 6C).

Mucous cysts

Mucous cysts commonly are associated with IP joint arthritis. Although the cause of mucous cysts remains controversial, nearly all published reports agree that these lesions are associated with some degree of osteoarthrosis affecting the underlying joint [30,31]. The lesion typically is localized to one side of the midline over the dorsal distal thumb (Fig. 7). Associated longitudinal grooving of the nail may be noted (Fig. 8). Patients who present with mucous cysts predominantly are female, most commonly in the fifth through seventh decades of life [32]. Apart from the cosmetic deformity, patients who have mucous cysts may complain of chronic drainage, recurrent infections, or persistent pain.

Mucous cyst excision with concomitant débridement of the underlying IP joint osteophyte currently is the most commonly accepted treatment [33–35]. In 1973, Eaton and colleagues [36] noted in their series of 44 patients that cyst excision with osteophyte débridement resulted in only one recurrence with complete disappearance of preoperative nail deformities within 6 months of surgery.

For excision of large mucous cysts, an extended dorsal advancement flap can minimize the risk for flap necrosis [37]. The broader flap also permits greater skin coverage distally, which can be helpful particularly after excision of large cysts. Planning the flap depends on the site of the mucous cyst. Ulnar-sided cysts, for example, are best served with a flap that is elevated from ulnar to radial for optimal coverage (Fig. 9). After application of a tourniquet, the cyst is removed

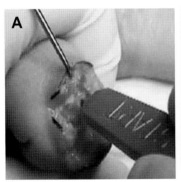
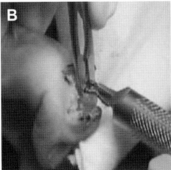
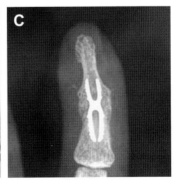

Fig. 6. The X-Fuse system (Memometal, Inc., Memphis, TN) allows for intramedullary placement of an implant for interphalangeal joint fusion. (*A*) Rasps of increasing size are used. (*B*) Once the trial implant has been placed, positioning is confirmed under fluoroscopic visualization. (*C*) Postoperative radiograph demonstrating a healed fusion.

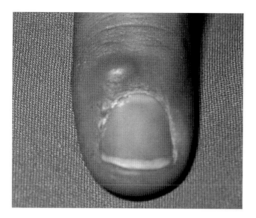

Fig. 7. Mucous cyst in the thumb. Note its position to one side of the midline. (*From* Shin EK, Jupiter JB. Flap advancement coverage after excision of large mucous cysts. Tech Hand Up Extrem Surg 2007;11:159–62.)

with a small ellipse of skin. The flap then is raised to the midaxial line on the opposite side, avoiding injury to the extensor peritenon (Fig. 10). The proximal extent of the flap depends on the amount of coverage required to permit a tension-free closure. The dorsal capsule and synovium are débrided to prevent cyst recurrence (Fig. 11). Care must be taken during dissection to avoid injury to the germinal nail matrix, which could result in postoperative nail deformity. The flap is advanced distally into the defect and closed with 4-0 nonabsorbable sutures.

Outcomes

Although MCP arthrodesis typically is the mainstay of treatment of arthritic thumbs, MCP

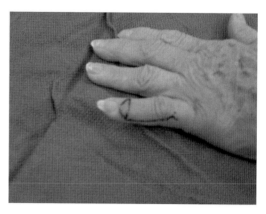

Fig. 9. Planning the flap depends upon the site of the mucous cyst. Ulnar-sided cysts are best served with a flap that is elevated from ulnar to radial for optimal coverage. The cyst is removed with an ellipse of skin. (*From* Shin EK, Jupiter JB. Flap advancement coverage after excision of large mucous cysts. Tech Hand Up Extrem Surg 2007;11:159–62; with permission.)

arthroplasty procedures demonstrate promise. The Steffee arthroplasty system was evaluated in 54 thumbs for long-term outcomes and implant survivorship [21]. Most of the patients included in this study underwent MCP joint arthroplasty for rheumatoid arthritis. Nevertheless, all patients demonstrated improvements in pain levels with an average follow-up period of 57 months. The average motion at the MCP joint was 21° (range 0° to 40°). Complications included a periprosthetic fracture, two late infections, and one gross loosening of the implant. The implant demonstrated 93% survivorship at 5 years and 89% survivorship at 10 years, with only four failures in 54 thumbs.

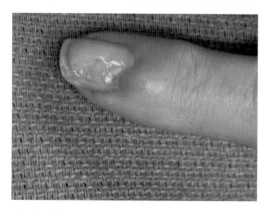

Fig. 8. Mucous cysts may cause significant nail ridging. (*From* Shin EK, Jupiter JB. Flap advancement coverage after excision of large mucous cysts. Tech Hand Up Extrem Surg 2007;11:159–62.)

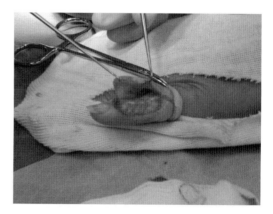

Fig. 10. The flap is raised, avoiding injury to the extensor mechanism. (*From* Shin EK, Jupiter JB. Flap advancement coverage after excision of large mucous cysts. Tech Hand Up Extrem Surg 2007;11:159–62.)

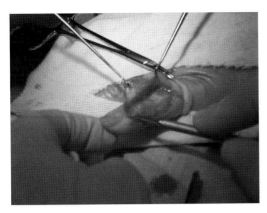

Fig. 11. The dorsal capsule and synovium are debrided to prevent cyst recurrence. (*From* Shin EK, Jupiter JB. Flap advancement coverage after excision of large mucous cysts. Tech Hand Up Extrem Surg 2007;11:159–62; with permission.)

No study, to the authors' knowledge, has examined the efficacy or survivorship of pyrocarbon implants in the thumb. Parker and colleagues [38] presented their preliminary findings with nonconstrained pyrocarbon implants in a retrospective review. Of the 142 MCP arthroplasties performed in 61 patients, 15 presented with primary osteoarthritis and three with posttraumatic arthritis. All arthroplasties were performed in the index, middle, ring, and small fingers. According to the analog pain scale, pain decreased from 73.0 to 8.5 of 100 with an average follow-up period of 17 months. The arc of motion improved from 44° to 58°. Radiographs at 1 year demonstrated stable prostheses in all osteoarthritis patients. From the short-term results reported, the investigators concluded that pyrocarbon arthroplasty provides good pain relief, patient satisfaction, and functional improvement in managing osteoarthritis.

Fusion rates for MCP arthrodesis typically are good. Stanley and colleagues [39] reviewed 42 cases of MCP arthrodesis and judged 83% of operations to be successful, with seven cases of pain or instability at the site of fusion (17%). Schmidt and colleagues [40] described a technique of thumb MCP joint arthrodesis using a 3.0-mm partially threaded cannulated screw and threaded washer (Synthes, Paoli, Pennsylvania) (Fig. 12). In 26 patients, the investigators found a 96% rate of fusion clinically and radiographically. The average time to radiographic union was 10 weeks with no infections and no requirements for hardware removal.

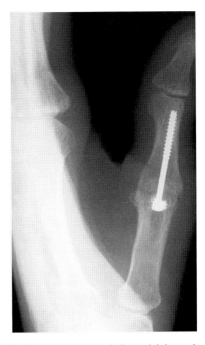

Fig. 12. Thumb metacarpophalangeal joint arthrodesis using a single 3.0 mm cannulated screw with threaded washer (Synthes, Paoli, PA). (*From* Schmidt CC, Zimmer SM, Boles SD. Arthrodesis of the thumb metacarpophalangeal joint using a cannulated screw and threaded washer. J Hand Surg [Am] 2004;29:1044–50; with permission.)

The major disadvantages of MCP joint arthrodesis include loss of precision mobility and increased stress placed on adjacent joints, resulting in progression of disease at the CMC and IP articulations. Despite these shortcomings, however, the authors continue to use MCP joint arthrodesis as the mainstay of treatment of moderate type deformities in active patients who require strong and stable thumbs.

The Indiana Hand Center experience with small joint arthrodesis was reviewed by Leibovic and Strickland [41]. In this series, Kirschner wires were associated with a 21% nonunion rate, tension bands with a 4.5% nonunion rate, and Herbert screws (Zimmer, Warsaw, Indiana) with a 0% nonunion rate. In contrast, Stern and Fulton [42] found that DIP nonunion rates were 11% to 12% despite the technique used. The techniques compared included crossed Kirschner wires (111 joints), interfragmentary wires and longitudinal Kirschner wires (43 joints), and Herbert screws (27 joints). There were 21 nonunions, of which 13 were pain free and six required subsequent arthrodesis. Twenty percent of the fused joints had major complications: nonunion, malunion, deep infection, and osteomyelitis (Fig. 13). Sixteen percent developed minor complications, such as superficial wound infections, dorsal skin necrosis, cold intolerance, proximal IP stiffness, paresthesias, and prominent hardware. Similarly, Brutus and colleagues [43] retrospectively reviewed their outcomes in 27 DIP or thumb IP joint arthrodeses using the Mini-Acutrak screw (Acumed, Beaverton, Oregon). Twenty-three of the 27 arthrodeses (85%) achieved bony union.

Uhl and Schneider [44] reviewed 76 consecutive cases of tension band arthrodeses in 63 patients. Follow-up in this series ranged from 6 to 38 months. The average time to radiographic union was 12 weeks. Only one joint failed to fuse but developed a stable, asymptomatic nonunion. The overall fusion rate was 99%. IJsselstein and colleagues [45] performed a retrospective review of 203 arthrodeses to compare percutaneous Kirschner wires with tension band fixation. In the Kirschner wire group, 18% of the patients had pin tract infections and in 15% re-arthrodeses were necessary. In the tension band group, 2% of the patients had an infection and in 5% re-arthrodeses were performed. In their hands, tension bands offered the best results.

Several complications have been reported after excision of mucous cysts. Fritz and colleagues [46] followed 86 mucous cysts in 79 patients who had an average follow-up of 2.6 years. Postoperative complications included loss of IP joint extension, superficial infection, swelling, pain, and numbness. Cyst recurrence was noted in only 3% of patients. Although preoperative nail deformities resolved in 15 of 25 digits (60%), four digits developed a nail deformity that was not present before surgery. If a patient continues to have pain after surgery with radiographic evidence of IP joint osteoarthritis, arthrodesis may be indicated for a later time.

Summary

The causes of primary osteoarthritis affecting the thumb MCP and IP articulations are poorly understood. Secondary causes of osteoarthritis include traumatic injury, soft tissue instability, infection, and congenital deformity. A high index of suspicion should be maintained for the presentation of gout. A thorough history and physical examination should include an assessment of the entire upper extremity with special attention to functional deficits with activities of daily living. A patient's ambulatory status also may be important in determining appropriate surgical care. Conservative therapies include NSAIDs, splint immobilization, activity modifications, and possibly corticosteroid injections. Patients who fail conservative treatments may benefit from surgical intervention in the form of arthroscopic synovectomy, arthroplasty, and arthrodesis. Treatment of mucous cysts tends to be conservative unless there is skin breakdown or nail ridging. Excision of mucous cysts with débridement of the IP articulation generally leads to good outcomes with low recurrence rates.

Arthroscopic synovectomy and joint replacement may play a useful role in the treatment of MCP joint arthritis. Such measures would preserve motion at the joint and possibly prevent the development of arthritic changes at the adjacent joints. Sufficient long-term studies of these treatments, however, have yet to be presented. Arthrodesis of the thumb MCP and IP joints is a successful and time-tested treatment. Fusion rates are between 83% and 100%. The technique for arthrodesis may play an important role in determining if fusion is successful, but several studies suggest that the actual technique used may be irrelevant.

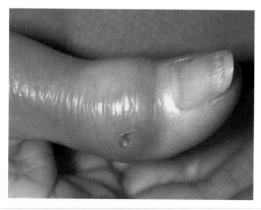

Fig. 13. Deep infection following attempted thumb interphalangeal joint arthrodesis using a headless compression screw.

References

[1] Peyron JG. The epidemiology of osteoarthritis. In: Moskowitz RW, Howell DS, Goldberg VM, et al, editors. Osteoarthritis: diagnosis and management. Philadelphia: WB Saunders; 1984. p. 9–27.

[2] Carr MM, Freiberg A. Osteoarthritis of the thumb: clinical aspects and management. Am Fam Physician 1994;50:995–1000.

[3] Xu L, Strauch RJ, Ateshian GA, et al. Topography of the osteoarthritic thumb carpometacarpal joint and its variations with regard to gender, age, site, and osteoarthritic stage. J Hand Surg [Am] 1998;23:454–64.

[4] Ateshian GA, Rosenwasser MP, Mow VC. Curvature characteristics and congruence of the thumb carpometacarpal joint: differences between female and male joints. J Biomech 1992;25:591–607.

[5] Fontana L, Neel S, Claise JM, et al. Osteoarthritis of the thumb carpometacarpal joint in women and occupational risk factors: a case-control study. J Hand Surg [Am] 2007;32:459–65.

[6] Feldon P, Belsky MR. Degenerative diseases of the metacarpophalangeal joints. Hand Clin 1987;3:429–47.

[7] Hunter DJ, Zhang Y, Nevitt MC, et al. Chopstick arthropathy: the Beijing osteoarthritis study. Arthritis Rheum 2004;50:1495–500.

[8] Lane NE, Bloch DA, Jones HH, et al. Osteoarthritis in the hand: a comparison of handedness and hand use. J Rheumatol 1989;16:637–42.

[9] Acheson RM, Chan YK, Clemett AR. New Haven survey of joint diseases. Distribution and symptoms of osteoarthrosis in the hands with reference to handedness. Ann Rheum Dis 1970;29:275–86.

[10] Roubenoff R, Klag MJ, Mead LA, et al. Incidence and risk factors for gout in white men. JAMA 1991;266:3004–7.

[11] Hume MC, Gellman H, McKellop H, et al. Functional range of motion of the joints of the hand. J Hand Surg [Am] 1990;15:240–3.

[12] Brooks PM. Nonsteroidal antiinflammatory drugs—differences and similarities. N Engl J Med 1991;324:1716–25.

[13] Bradley JD. Comparison of an antiinflammatory dose of ibuprofen, an analgesic dose of ibuprofen, and acetaminophen in the treatment of patients with osteoarthritis of the knee. N Engl J Med 1991;325:87–91.

[14] Sahi SP, Basu SK, Bansal SK. Nonsteroidal antiinflammatory drugs and gastrointestinal bleeding in the elderly. Br J Clin Pract 1990;44:22–3.

[15] Roth S. Misoprostol heals gastroduodenal injury in patients with rheumatoid arthritis receiving aspirin. Arch Intern Med 1989;149:775–9.

[16] Rozental TD, Sculco TP. Intra-articular corticosteroids: an updated overview. Am J Orthop 2000;29:18–23.

[17] Pelletier JP. The therapeutic effects of NSAIDs and corticosteroids in osteoarthritis: to be or not to be. J Rheumatol 1989;16:266–9.

[18] Badia A. Arthroscopy of the trapeziometacarpal and metacarpophalangeal joints. J Hand Surg [Am] 2007;32:707–24.

[19] Earp BE, Leung AC, Blazar PE, et al. Arthroscopic hemitrapeziectomy with tendon interposition for arthritis at the first carpometacarpal joint. Tech Hand Up Extrem Surg 2008;12:38–42.

[20] Beckenbaugh RD, Steffee A. Total joint arthroplasty for the metacarpophalangeal joint of the thumb—a preliminary report. Orhtopaedics 1981;4:295–8.

[21] McGovern RM, Shin AY, Beckenbaugh RD, et al. Long-term results of cemented Stefee arthroplasty of the thumb metacarpophalangeal joint. J Hand Surg [Am] 2001;26:115–22.

[22] Bicknell RT, MacDermid J, Roth JH. Assessment of thumb metacarpophalangeal joint arthrodesis using a single longitudinal K-wire. J Hand Surg [Am] 2007;32:677–84.

[23] Messer TM, Nagle DJ, Martinez AG. Thumb metacarpophalangeal joint arthrodesis using the AO 3.0-mm cannulated screw: surgical technique. J Hand Surg [Am] 2002;27:910–2.

[24] Carroll RE, Hill NA. Small joint arthrodesis in hand reconstruction. J Bone Joint Surg Am 1969;51:1219–21.

[25] Inglis AE, Hamlin C, Sengelmann R, et al. Reconstruction of the metacarpophalangeal joint of the thumb in rheumatoid arthritis. J Bone Joint Surg [Am] 1972;54:704–12.

[26] Swanson AB, Herndon JH. Flexible (silicone) implant arthrolasty of the metacarpophalangeal joint of the thumb. J Bone Joint Surg Am 1977;59:362–8.

[27] Katzman SS, Gibeault JD, Dickson K, et al. Use of a Herbert screw for interphalangeal joint arthrodesis. Clin Orthop Relat Res 1993;296:127–32.

[28] Leibovic SJ. Arthrodesis of the interphalangeal joints with headless compression screws. J Hand Surg [Am] 2007;32:1113–9.

[29] Wyrsch B, Dawson J, Aufranc S, et al. Distal interphalangeal joint arthrodesis comparing tension-band wire and herbert screw: a biomechanical and dimensional analysis. J Hand Surg [Am] 1996;21:438–43.

[30] Constant E, Royer JR, Pollard RJ, et al. Mucous cysts of the fingers. Plast Reconstr Surg 1969;43:241–6.

[31] Kleinert HE, Kutz JE, Fishman JH, et al. Etiology and treatment of the so-called mucous cyst of the finger. J Bone Joint Surg Am 1972;54:1455–8.

[32] Nelson CL, Sawmiller S, Phalen GS. Ganglions of the wrist and hand. J Bone Joint Surg Am 1972;54:1459–64.

[33] Crawford RJ, Gupta A, Risitano G, et al. Mucous cyst excision of the distal interphalangeal joint: treatment by simple excision or excision and rotation flap. J Hand Surg [Br] 1990;15:113–4.

[34] Dodge LD, Brown RL, Niebauer JJ, et al. The treatment of mucous cysts: long-term follow-up in sixty-two cases. J Hand Surg [Am] 1984;9:901–4.

[35] Kasdan ML, Stallings SP, Leis VM, et al. Outcome of surgically treated mucous cysts of the hand. J Hand Surg [Am] 1994;19:504–7.

[36] Eaton RG, Dobranski AI, Littler JW. Marginal osteophyte excision in treatment of mucous cysts. J Bone Joint Surg Am 1973;55:570–4.

[37] Shin EK, Jupiter JB. Flap advancement coverage after excision of large mucous cysts. Tech Hand Up Extrem Surg 2007;11:159–62.

[38] Parker WL, Rizzo M, Moran SL, et al. Preliminary results of nonconstrained pyrolytic carbon arthroplasty for metacarpophalangeal joint arthritis. J Hand Surg [Am] 2007;32:1496–505.

[39] Stanley JK, Smith EJ, Muirhead AG. Arthrodesis of the metacarpophalangeal joint of the thumb: a review of 42 cases. J Hand Surg [Br] 1989;14:291–3.

[40] Schmidt CC, Zimmer SM, Boles SD. Arthrodesis of the thumb metacarpophalangeal joint using a cannulated screw and threaded washer. J Hand Surg [Am] 2004;29:1044–50.

[41] Leibovic SJ, Strickland JW. Arthrodesis of the proximal interphalangeal joint of the finger: comparison of the use of the Jerbert screw with other fixation methods. J Hand Surg [Am] 1994;19:181–8.

[42] Stern PJ, Fulton DB. Distal interphalangeal joint arthrodesis: an analysis of complications. J Hand Surg [Am] 1992;17:1139–45.

[43] Brutus JP, Palmer AK, Mosher JF, et al. Use of a headless compressive screw for distal interphalangeal joint arthrodesis in digits: clinical outcome and review of complications. J Hand Surg [Am] 2006;31:85–9.

[44] Uhl RL, Schneider LH. Tension band arthrodesis of finger joints: a retrospective review of 76 consecutive cases. J Hand Surg [Am] 1992;17:518–22.

[45] IJsselstein CB, van Egmond DB, Hovius SE, et al. Results of small-joint arthrodesis: comparison of Kirschner wire fixation with tension band wire technique. J Hand Surg [Am] 1992;17:952–6.

[46] Fritz GR, Stern PJ, Dickey M. Complications following mucous cyst excision. J Hand Surg [Br] 1997;22:222–5.

ELSEVIER
SAUNDERS

Hand Clin 24 (2008) 251–261

HAND
CLINICS

Early Treatment of Degenerative Arthritis of the Thumb Carpometacarpal Joint

Jeffrey Yao, MD[a,*], Min J. Park, MMSc[b,c]

[a]Robert A. Chase Hand and Upper Limb Center, Department of Orthopedic Surgery,
Stanford University Hospitals and Clinics, 770 Welch Road, Suite 400, Palo Alto, CA 94304, USA
[b]Department of Orthopedic Surgery, Hospital of the University of Pennsylvania, 3400 Spruce Street,
2 Silverstein, Philadelphia, PA 19104, USA
[c]Department of Orthopedic Surgery, Rhode Island Hospital, Warren Alpert Medical School
of Brown University, Providence, RI 02905, USA

The thumb carpometacarpal (CMC) joint is complex and subjected to constant loading stresses in multiple directions. Several ligaments surround the joint, the strongest and most important being the palmar oblique or "beak" ligament. These ligaments form a capsule that stabilizes the joint [1]. Degenerative arthritis of the thumb CMC joint is not an uncommon condition, particularly in postmenopausal women [2]. The age-adjusted prevalence of CMC arthritis based on radiographic evidence has been reported to be 15% for the female population and 7% for the male population [3]. The prevalence increases to 33% for the postmenopausal female population [2]. The wide range of motion, including abduction/adduction, flexion/extension, and axial rotation, contributes to the high prevalence of thumb CMC degenerative arthritis, more so than in other joints [4,5]. Many investigators have attempted to establish the causal relationships between predisposing factors and thumb CMC arthritis. The condition may be acquired due to various underlying medical conditions, acute or chronic trauma, advanced age, hormonal factors, various different shapes of individual joints, and genetic influences [6]. There is a report correlating obesity to thumb CMC arthritis as well [7]. Occupational factors are also believed to have a role in the development of thumb CMC arthritis, but the results seem to be inconclusive at best, and it has been difficult to establish a direct correlation between the disease process and any particular occupation [8–10].

Presentation and classification

Regardless of the etiology, there is no debate that degenerative arthritis of the thumb CMC joint is a common treatable condition. Over the years, many different diagnostic methods have been established. History provided by the patient including pain with pinching and gripping activities without any significant evidence of trauma is common. Difficulty turning keys, opening jars, and gripping doorknobs is classic. Physical examination should be focused on the dorsoradial aspect of the wrist. Pertinent findings to rule out other entities in the differential diagnosis, such as de Quervain's tenosynovitis, flexor carpi radialis tendonitis, extensor carpi radialis longus/extensor carpi radialis brevis tendonitis, scaphoid pathology, and scaphotrapeziotrapezoid pathology, should be sought. Similarly, stenosing flexor tenosynovitis (trigger thumb) and carpal tunnel syndrome may present as basilar thumb pain and must be ruled out. Of the diagnostic classification methods, the radiographic staging method established by Eaton and Littler [11] is the most popularly used. Although individual symptoms may not correlate with the Eaton diagnostic criteria, the radiographic findings provide insight into whether a patient would truly benefit from more conservative treatment options. In the past, early

* Corresponding author.
  E-mail address: jyao@stanford.edu (J. Yao).

stages of thumb CMC arthritis were treated mainly with nonoperative modalities, but recently there has been increasing interest in early surgical options as well. With the use of nonoperative treatment options and the relatively less invasive surgical options, patients may be able to avoid more significant procedures, experience faster pain relief, and achieve better thumb function in their activities of daily living more quickly.

Nonoperative treatments

Activity modification

One of the key elements of nonoperative treatment of thumb CMC arthritis is pain control. Because the functional level of patients tends to be inversely related to their pain level [12], improving levels of pain may significantly help patients with activities of daily living. Patient education toward modifying daily activity to effectively rest the thumb is an important consideration for any stage of treatment. Learning to avoid inflammatory activities of the thumb, such as pinching, gripping, lifting, and twisting, may greatly improve a patient's symptoms, especially in an acutely flared thumb. Also, by dividing stress among multiple joints or using assistive devices, patients may increase their function significantly without further damaging their thumb CMC joint [12]. Patients are often encouraged to understand the principles behind activity modification and the assistive devices, and to help lose the habits that may place excessive load on the thumb CMC joint over a long period of time [13]. When implemented correctly, patient education regarding joint protection is shown to improve grip strength and pain relief [13,14]. Strengthening and flexibility exercises are only recommended for patients who have early stage disease without significant pain and inflammation [12]. When appropriate, abduction combined with slight medial rotation and flexion of the thumb CMC joint increases the stability at the base of the joint. Strengthening exercises should focus on training the thenar eminence, the abductor pollicis longus, and the extensor pollicis longus to counter the flexion-adduction forces of the adductor pollicis muscle. These measures potentially prevent the adduction contracture with loss of the first web space [15,16].

Medication

Non-steroidal anti-inflammatory drugs (NSAIDs) are the most frequently used pain control medications. They reduce inflammation, synovitis, and pain, but there is no evidence that these medications actually stop or reverse the disease process. Because there is essentially no difference in the effectiveness of currently available NSAIDs in terms of pain control in arthritis [17], the decision to use one medication over another should be based on other patient factors. Although NSAIDs may be part of any patient's treatment regimen, one should be cognizant that the medications will not stop or reverse the progression of disease.

Splinting

The use of splints has been proven to give pain relief and potentially delay disease progression. Splinting alone, leading to "forced rest" of the thumb with resulting decreased synovitis, may be beneficial to patients with early stage thumb CMC arthritis [18]. The goals of splinting the thumb CMC joint are to increase stability, reduce pain, decrease inflammation, improve function, and reduce mechanical stress that may be causing the instability. Patients with unstable or hypermobile thumb CMC joints are good candidates for wearing splints. The splint should induce palmar abduction and incorporate slight flexion and medial rotation. This position helps with preservation of the first web space and also increases the natural stability of the joint by increasing the fitting of the joint surface [12].

The wrist-CMC immobilization splint, also known as the long opponens splint, has been available for a long time. This splint supports both the wrist and hand and immobilizes the wrist in about 10 to 20 degrees of extension, the CMC joint in relative palmar abduction, and the metacarpophalangeal (MCP) joint in about 30 degrees of flexion. The interphalangeal joint remains free. This configuration shifts the center of pressure within the CMC joint dorsally. This shift effectively unloads the palmar side of the CMC joint, relieving the area susceptible to degenerative changes [19,20]. The short opponens splint, also known as CMC-MCP immobilization splint or hand-based thumb spica splint, is similar to the long opponens splint, but the wrist is not immobilized (Fig. 1A,B). A modified short opponens splint is also available that maintains the CMC joint in near extension while allowing the MCP joint free flexion and extension [21]. These splints are commercially available or may be custom fitted out of a malleable plastic such as thermoplast.

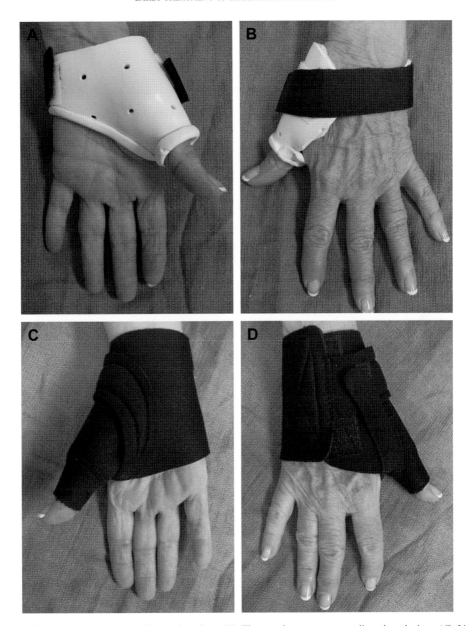

Fig. 1. (*A*) Thermoplast opponens splint, volar view. (*B*) Thermoplast opponens splint, dorsal view. (*C*) Neoprene opponens splint, volar view. (*D*) Neoprene opponens splint, dorsal view.

It is the authors' preference to use custom-fitted splints made by our therapists because we believe they are more individualized as well as more rigid, providing increased stabilization.

The effectiveness of the various splints has been shown in early stages of thumb CMC joint arthritis. Although the long opponens splint and the short opponens splint are comparable in terms of pain relief, patients tend to prefer the short opponens splint because of its less bulky design [18]. Similarly, neoprene splints (Fig. 1C,D) may be used for daily use while a more rigid splint is used at night, improving patient compliance. The authors are currently evaluating the effectiveness of these less intrusive, but potentially less stabilizing splints when compared with stiffer splints long term. The benefits of splinting, regardless of the design, should be achieved by 3 to 4 weeks from the initiation of therapy.

Injections

When activity modification, NSAIDs, and splinting fail to provide necessary pain relief, one may consider corticosteroid injections into the thumb CMC joint. The primary goal of the corticosteroid injection is to reduce inflammation and achieve pain relief, much like the use of NSAIDs. This intra-articular injection may provide short-term pain relief, but its long-term effect for relieving symptoms is questionable [22,23]. It has been shown that corticosteroid injections, along with splinting, may provide symptom relief for patients with Eaton stage I disease, but no such benefit has been reported in moderate-to-severe cases of thumb CMC arthritis [24]. The authors' preference is to provide the injection only for patients in whom the diagnosis is somewhat unclear as a diagnostic as well as therapeutic modality, or for patients who wish to delay surgical intervention in the short term. Our usual cocktail to be injected consists of 0.7 mL of 1% lidocaine without epinephrine with 0.7 mL of betamethasone (Celestone, 6 mg/mL) solution injected into the joint. We prefer betamethasone due to its water solubility and because it does not tend to leave intra-articular precipitate deposits; however, several commercially available corticosteroids are acceptable for use in the CMC joint.

The patient's thumb CMC joint is palpated while the thumb is adducted and abducted. The injection is given with a 25-gauge needle just proximal to the radial base of the thumb metacarpal, radial and volar to the extensor pollicis brevis tendon. The needle should be angled distally and advanced until it penetrates the joint capsule. Providers should use corticosteroid injections sparingly, because they may accelerate cartilage loss and exacerbate capsular attenuation [25].

There has been increasing interest in the use of hyaluronic acid preparations stemming from their use in the knee joint. Hyaluronic acid is thought to act as a lubricant and contribute to joint homeostasis [26]. Investigators have shown that intra-articular injections of hyaluronic acid into knee joints augment the flow of synovial fluid, normalize the synthesis, inhibit the degradation of endogenous hyaluronic acid, and bring pain relief to patients [27–29]. With their apparent efficacy in the knee joint, several investigators have attempted the injection of hyaluronic acid into thumb CMC joints. Although the reports seem to indicate that hyaluronic acid preparations do confer some benefits similar to that of corticosteroid injections, there is no definitive evidence that hyaluronic acid preparations are as effective or superior to corticosteroid injection [30–33]. Larger scale studies with longer follow-up periods are necessary to determine the efficacy of hyaluronic acid injections into the thumb CMC joint long term.

Traditional surgical approaches to thumb carpometacarpal arthritis

Many surgical techniques are available for the treatment of thumb CMC arthritis that is refractory to conservative nonsurgical measures. These techniques are briefly mentioned herein for reference and are described in greater detail elsewhere in this issue.

Although thumb CMC joint arthrodesis may achieve excellent joint stability, it is associated with loss of motion and transfer of the load and stress to neighboring joints [34,35]. Since its introduction, ligament reconstruction and tendon interposition (LRTI) has been favored by many hand surgeons because early synthetic implants were thought to be unreliable [36]. Silicone implants, in particular, are associated with implant instability or subluxation in 25% of cases [37]. Understanding the role of the palmar oblique (beak) ligament in the pathophysiology of osteoarthritis at the thumb CMC joint further supports the concept of ligament reconstruction [20]. Nevertheless, some authorities have recently questioned the necessity of the ligament reconstruction portion of LRTI [38], and the development of more reliable new materials has provided greater options in terms of managing thumb CMC joint arthritis [39,40].

Total joint arthroplasty, much like total hip arthroplasty, using a bone cement technique is a safe and reliable technique for patients with Eaton stage III and early stage IV disease [41]; however, aseptic loosening of the implant is a common complication, and there have been reports questioning the long-term stability of the implants [42,43]. These implants have failed to garner widespread support thus far. Although simple trapeziectomy was described quite some time ago [44], there is a renewed interest in the technique. Study of the hematoma distraction arthroplasty has shown equal or better long-term, follow-up results when compared with other more traditional techniques [45]. A recent independent meta-analysis identified simple trapeziectomy as the preferable technique for treatment of advanced thumb CMC arthritis [46]. Although the surgeon's comfort and the patient's preference influence which arthroplasty technique is used, most of these techniques are invasive and require prolonged recovery time. These options are appropriate for moderate-to-severe stages (Eaton stages III-IV) but may be excessive for patients with moderate symptoms or an early stage of the disease process.

Surgical intervention for early stage arthritis of the thumb carpometacarpal

Abduction-extension osteotomy

For the patient who fails a full course of conservative management and still presents with early stage thumb CMC joint arthritis, there are several less invasive surgical treatment options. In fact, some authorities believe that progressive loss of cartilage is inevitable once there is evidence of thumb CMC arthritis, and suggest that early surgical intervention would ultimately benefit patients [25]. The abduction-extension osteotomy is a simple technique that is not frequently used. It is useful in a small subset of younger patients with early stage disease [47]. Because thumb CMC joint arthritis is associated with degeneration of the palmar beak ligament and neighboring joint surface, shifting the joint load from the palmar cartilage to the dorsal surface with the osteotomy may provide lasting pain relief, reverse the adduction contracture, and improve grip and pinch strength [48,49]. Although the osteotomy technique can provide excellent results, it is not appropriate for patients with advanced disease in whom the dorsal joint surface is already involved. The recovery following this technique is also prolonged given the immobilization necessary to heal the osteotomy.

Arthroscopy

With the development of fine arthroscopic instruments, hand surgeons are currently interested in using arthroscopic techniques for patients with thumb CMC arthritis. Patients with early (Eaton stage I) disease may benefit from arthroscopic debridement, synovectomy, and capsulorrhaphy [50]. There is an arthroscopic classification of thumb trapeziometacarpal osteoarthritis as well [25]. Stage I of the classification indicates intact articular cartilage with disruption of the

dorsoradial ligament and diffuse synovial hypertrophy, along with inconsistent attenuation of the anterior oblique ligament. In stage II, frank eburnation of the articular cartilage at the ulnar third of the base of the first metacarpal and central third of the distal surface of the trapezium is observed, along with disruption of the dorsoradial ligament and increased synovial hypertrophy. Further attenuation of the anterior oblique ligament is observed in stage II as well. By stage III, widespread, full-thickness cartilage loss with or without a peripheral rim on both articular surfaces can be observed, with less severe synovitis. The volar ligaments are frayed, and significant laxity is detected [25].

The authors' treatment algorithm for early thumb CMC arthritis (Eaton stages I-III) refractory to conservative measures involves thumb CMC arthroscopy, hemitrapeziectomy, and Kirschner wire fixation, with or without interposition. The rare young laborer who has early arthritis may benefit from the extension-abduction osteotomy. Only patients with Eaton stage IV (pantrapezial) disease would have an open procedure, giving patients with early stage disease less invasive alternatives to traditional open techniques.

Surgical technique

The arthroscopic technique may be performed under regional (preferred) or general anesthesia. Regional anesthesia is recommended for immediate postoperative pain relief. The standard wrist arthroscopy tower and equipment with the 2.3-mm arthroscope is used for the procedure. The thumb is placed alone in a finger trap and hung from the tower at approximately 5 to 10 pounds of longitudinal traction. A sterile elastic bandage (Coban, 3M, St. Paul, Minnesota) is wrapped around the finger trap for stability and also around the hand and the tower to stabilize the hand outside of the operative field. The thumb CMC joint is found by palpating proximally along the thumb metacarpal until a depression is felt. At this level, the 1-R (radial to the abductor pollicis longus tendon) and 1-U (ulnar to the extensor pollicis brevis tendon) portals are marked (Fig. 2) [1,51]. The arm tourniquet is placed as proximally in the axilla as possible and inflated to 250 mm Hg. Normal saline in a syringe is injected into the thumb CMC joint via either portal to insufflate the joint and confirm the portal location and angle of entry. A No. 11 scalpel is used to incise only the skin of the 1-U portal. A blunt mosquito clamp is

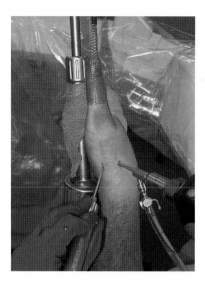

Fig. 2. The arthroscope in the 1-U portal and the shaver in the 1-R portal.

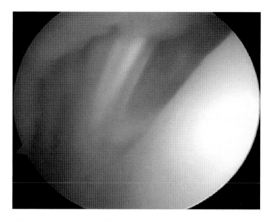

Fig. 3. Anterior oblique beak ligament viewed from the 1-U portal. Trapezium is shown on the right side of the image and the thumb metacarpal on the top of the image.

then used to gently spread down to the level of the CMC joint capsule to minimize the potential of injuring the neighboring abductor pollicis longus, extensor pollicis brevis, and extensor pollicis longus tendons and branches of the dorsal radial sensory nerve and radial artery.

Once the joint is entered, the injected saline should egress, and the 2.3-mm arthroscope is inserted. We prefer constant saline inflow via the arthroscopy pump set to 60 mm Hg to provide adequate joint distention for visualization and irrigation of fragments. Diagnostic arthroscopy is performed, and the 1-R portal is made under direct visualization and using the same atraumatic technique. The dorsoradial, posterior oblique, and ulnar collateral ligament are seen best with the arthroscope in the 1-R portal. The volar/anterior oblique beak ligament is best visualized via the 1-U portal (Fig. 3) [1]. In an anatomic study, Walsh [52] describes a thenar portal that is approximately 90 degrees to the 1-U portal. This portal may be safer than the 1-R portal because it has been shown to be farther away from any potentially injured structures, such as branches of the radial sensory nerve. An 18-gauge localizing needle is introduced into the CMC joint through the thenar musculature under direct arthroscopic visualization. Once proper position of the needle is confirmed, the thenar portal is made in the same fashion as the other portals (Fig. 4). The fact that this portal is 90 degrees from the 1-U

portal may also make it more useful and easier to use during partial trapeziectomy with the arthroscope in the 1-U portal (Fig. 5).

A 3.5-mm, full-radius shaver is used via the thenar portal to debride any degenerative articular cartilage and synovium (Fig. 6). Often, loose bodies may be encountered in the joint. These bodies may be fixed to the surrounding soft tissue or floating freely and should be excised (Fig. 7). A 2.9-mm burr is then used to begin the

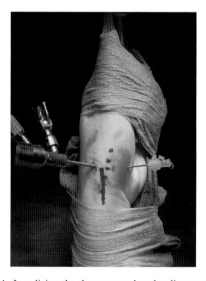

Fig. 4. Localizing the thenar portal under direct arthroscopic visualization with the use of an 18-gauge needle. Abductor pollicis longus and extensor pollicis brevis tendons are marked.

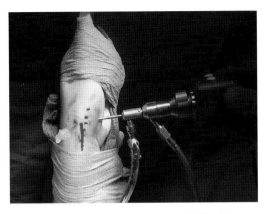

Fig. 5. Arthroscope in the thenar portal. The 18-gauge needle is in the 1-U portal for outflow.

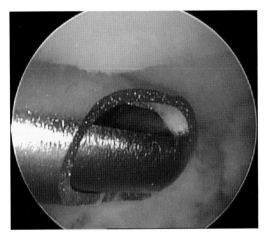

Fig. 6. The 3.5-mm full radius shaver is used to debride the soft tissue.

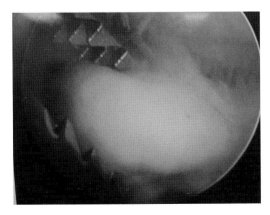

Fig. 7. Removal of a loose body using an arthroscopic grasper.

hemitrapeziectomy. Once enough space has been made between the metacarpal and the remaining trapezium, a larger, 3.5-mm burr may be used to complete the hemitrapeziectomy (Fig. 8). At least 3 to 5 mm of the distal trapezium should be excised. In cases of severe arthritis (Eaton stage IV) with pantrapezial changes where an open procedure was deferred, arthroscopy is still an option. The hemitrapezium is excised, the distal scaphoid is excised, and partial proximal trapezoidectomy is also performed.

It is often useful to use fluoroscopy to guide the level of resection and to identify any residual bone (Fig. 9). Alternating instruments and the arthroscope between the portals also helps in visualization and the complete resection of the hemitrapezium (Fig. 10).

Some patients present with concomitant ligamentous instability. It is essential to restore stability of the remaining CMC joint, especially following the hemitrapeziectomy. To aid in the restoration of this stability, an electrothermal radiofrequency probe is used for shrinkage of the ligaments (Fig. 11). This process serves to tighten the capsular ligaments, specifically the volar oblique beak ligament (Oratec Interventions, Menlo Park, California).

At this stage of the procedure, an interposition may be elected. Autograft (palmaris longus tendon) or prosthetic material (eg, Artelon spacer, a polycaprolactone-based polyurethane urea, Artimplant, Sweden) may be interposed into the newly formed space to assist in the prevention of proximal migration of the thumb metacarpal, based on surgeon preference (Fig. 12). The

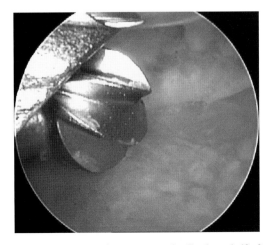

Fig. 8. The 3.5-mm burr removes the distal one half of the trapezium.

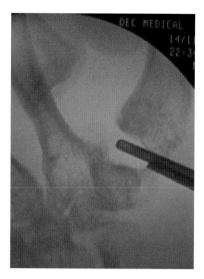

Fig. 9. Fluoroscopy aids in determining an adequate level of resection.

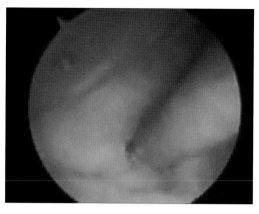

Fig. 11. A radiofrequency probe is used for electrothermal shrinkage of the capsular ligaments.

interposition material is inserted via the thenar portal and secured into place before wound closure.

In patients with significant MCP hyperextensibility (deformities greater than 20 degrees), either fusion or capsulodesis is performed to stabilize the joint. A 0.045-in Kirschner wire is then used to pin the thumb metacarpal to the residual trapezium or scaphoid in the reduced position with slight abduction to prevent proximal migration (Fig. 13).

The portals are closed with a 4-0 monofilament suture, and the patient is placed in a short arm thumb spica splint with adequate padding of the pin. The patient returns for follow-up 2 weeks postoperatively for suture removal and is placed in a short arm thumb spica thermoplast splint. At 4 weeks, the Kirschner wire is removed, and range of motion exercises are instituted.

Appropriate hand therapy is essential to the success of this procedure. Gentle active and active-assisted range of motion exercises are begun immediately following removal of the Kirschner wire. Another advantage of an arthroscopic approach is that there are no functional restrictions once the capsule has healed, and

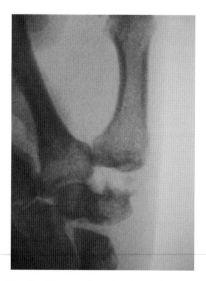

Fig. 10. The completed hemitrapeziectomy.

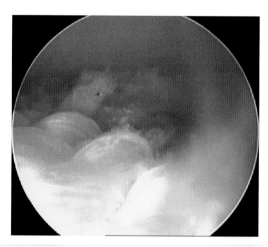

Fig. 12. An interposition spacer (Artelon) is placed in the newly created void. The metacarpal base is at the top of the image.

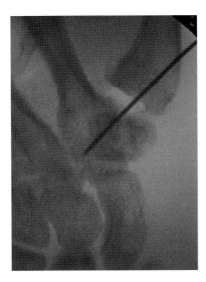

Fig. 13. A 0.045-in Kirschner wire is used to keep the metacarpal reduced. The wire is removed at the 4-week postoperative visit.

therapy progresses to strengthening exercises as the patient tolerates.

Results

In the authors' experience, 88% of the patients who had arthroscopic hemi- or complete trapeziectomy had a good-to-excellent outcome. Many patients seemed to prefer the arthroscopic procedure over the standard open procedure done on the contralateral side. Our current experience is comparable to that reported previously [53].

As is true in more common open procedures, potential complications of the arthroscopic technique include irritation or laceration of the dorsal radial sensory nerve, tendon laceration or rupture, and radial artery injury. We did not encounter any of these complications. Although the application of arthroscopic techniques for thumb CMC arthritis is a relatively new management strategy, our early results have been promising and should be explored further for additional application and improvement of the technique.

Summary

Because there is documented efficacy of available nonoperative management strategies, patients with early thumb CMC arthritis should be given an opportunity to go through a full course of nonoperative management, including activity modification, NSAIDs, splinting, therapy,

and corticosteroid injections. Splinting, in some cases, may actually reverse some of the early anatomic deformities sustained by patients [18]; however, once begun, thumb CMC arthritis will more likely be a progressive disease for which only surgical intervention may provide lasting pain relief and improvement in functional status. The emerging arthroscopic technique provides a safe, reliable option for patients who require surgical intervention early in the disease process.

References

[1] Berger RA. A technique for arthroscopic evaluation of the first carpometacarpal joint. J Hand Surg [Am] 1997;22:1077–80.

[2] Armstrong AL, Hunter JB, Davis TR. The prevalence of degenerative arthritis of the base of the thumb in postmenopausal women. J Hand Surg [Br] 1994;19:340–1.

[3] Haara MM, Heliovaara M, Kroger H, et al. Osteoarthritis in the carpometacarpal joint of the thumb: prevalence and associations with disability and mortality. J Bone Joint Surg Am 2004;86:1452–7.

[4] Barron OA, Glickel SZ, Eaton RG. Basal joint arthritis of the thumb. J Am Acad Orthop Surg 2000;8:314–23.

[5] Kuczynski K. Carpometacarpal joint of the human thumb. J Anat 1974;118:119–26.

[6] Cicuttini FM, Spector TD. The epidemiology of osteoarthritis of the hand. Rev Rhum Engl Ed 1995;62:3S–8S.

[7] Cicuttini FM, Baker JR, Spector TD. The association of obesity with osteoarthritis of the hand and knee in women: a twin study. J Rheumatol 1996;23:1221–6.

[8] Fontana L, Neel S, Claise JM, et al. Osteoarthritis of the thumb carpometacarpal joint in women and occupational risk factors: a case-control study. J Hand Surg [Am] 2007;32:459–65.

[9] Minuk GY, Waggoner JG, Hoofnagle JH, et al. Pipetter's thumb. N Engl J Med 1982;306:751.

[10] Turner WE. Pricers thumb. N Z Med J 1991;104:501–2.

[11] Eaton RG, Littler JW. Ligament reconstruction for the painful thumb carpometacarpal joint. J Bone Joint Surg Am 1973;55:1655–66.

[12] Neumann DA, Bielefeld T. The carpometacarpal joint of the thumb: stability, deformity, and therapeutic intervention. J Orthop Sports Phys Ther 2003;33:386–99.

[13] Hammond A, Freeman K. One-year outcomes of a randomized controlled trial of an educational-behavioural joint protection programme for people with rheumatoid arthritis. Rheumatology (Oxford) 2001;40:1044–51.

[14] Stamm TA, Machold KP, Smolen JS, et al. Joint protection and home hand exercises improve hand

function in patients with hand osteoarthritis: a randomized controlled trial. Arthritis Rheum 2002;47:44–9.

[15] Pellegrini VD Jr. Pathomechanics of the thumb trapeziometacarpal joint. Hand Clin 2001;17:175–84.

[16] Poole JU, Pellegrini VD Jr. Arthritis of the thumb basal joint complex. J Hand Ther 2000;13:91–107.

[17] Brooks PM, Day RO. Nonsteroidal anti-inflammatory drugs–differences and similarities. N Engl J Med 1991;324:1716–25.

[18] Weiss S, LaStayo P, Mills A, et al. Prospective analysis of splinting the first carpometacarpal joint: an objective, subjective, and radiographic assessment. J Hand Ther 2000;13:218–26.

[19] Moulton MJ, Parentis MA, Kelly MJ, et al. Influence of metacarpophalangeal joint position on basal joint-loading in the thumb. J Bone Joint Surg Am 2001;83:709–16.

[20] Pellegrini VD Jr. Osteoarthritis of the trapeziometacarpal joint: the pathophysiology of articular cartilage degeneration. I. Anatomy and pathology of the aging joint. J Hand Surg [Am] 1991;16:967–74.

[21] Colditz JC. The biomechanics of a thumb carpometacarpal immobilization splint: design and fitting. J Hand Ther 2000;13:228–35.

[22] Joshi R. Intra-articular corticosteroid injection for first carpometacarpal osteoarthritis. J Rheumatol 2005;32:1305–6.

[23] Meenagh GK, Patton J, Kynes C, et al. A randomised controlled trial of intra-articular corticosteroid injection of the carpometacarpal joint of the thumb in osteoarthritis. Ann Rheum Dis 2004;63:1260–3.

[24] Day CS, Gelberman R, Patel AA, et al. Basal joint osteoarthritis of the thumb: a prospective trial of steroid injection and splinting. J Hand Surg [Am] 2004;29:247–51.

[25] Badia A. Trapeziometacarpal arthroscopy: a classification and treatment algorithm. Hand Clin 2006;22:153–63.

[26] Laurent TC, Fraser JR. Hyaluronan. FASEB J 1992;6:2397–404.

[27] Peyron JG. Intra-articular hyaluronan injections in the treatment of osteoarthritis: state-of-the-art review. J Rheumatol Suppl 1993;39:10–5.

[28] Peyron JG. A new approach to the treatment of osteoarthritis: viscosupplementation. Osteoarthritis Cartilage 1993;1:85–7.

[29] Rydell N, Balazs EA. Effect of intra-articular injection of hyaluronic acid on the clinical symptoms of osteoarthritis and on granulation tissue formation. Clin Orthop Relat Res 1971;80:25–32.

[30] Roux C, Fontas E, Breuil V, et al. Injection of intra-articular sodium hyaluronidate (Sinovial) into the carpometacarpal joint of the thumb (CMC1) in osteoarthritis. A prospective evaluation of efficacy. Joint Bone Spine 2007;74:368–72.

[31] Fuchs S, Erbe T, Fischer HL, et al. Intra-articular hyaluronic acid versus glucocorticoid injections for nonradicular pain in the lumbar spine. J Vasc Interv Radiol 2005;16:1493–8.

[32] Fuchs S, Monikes R, Wohlmeiner A, et al. Intra-articular hyaluronic acid compared with corticoid injections for the treatment of rhizarthrosis. Osteoarthritis Cartilage 2006;14:82–8.

[33] Stahl S, Karsh-Zafrir I, Ratzon N, et al. Comparison of intra-articular injection of depot corticosteroid and hyaluronic acid for treatment of degenerative trapeziometacarpal joints. J Clin Rheumatol 2005;11:299–302.

[34] Damen A, van der Lei B, Robinson PH. Bilateral osteoarthritis of the trapeziometacarpal joint treated by bilateral tendon interposition arthroplasty. J Hand Surg [Br] 1997;22:96–9.

[35] Hartigan BJ, Stern PJ, Kiefhaber TR. Thumb carpometacarpal osteoarthritis: arthrodesis compared with ligament reconstruction and tendon interposition. J Bone Joint Surg Am 2001;83:1470–8.

[36] Tomaino MM, Pellegrini VD Jr, Burton RI. Arthroplasty of the basal joint of the thumb: long-term follow-up after ligament reconstruction with tendon interposition. J Bone Joint Surg Am 1995;77:346–55.

[37] Swanson AB, deGoot Swanson G, Watermeier JJ. Trapezium implant arthroplasty: long-term evaluation of 150 cases. J Hand Surg [Am] 1981;6:125–41.

[38] Kuhns CA, Meals RA. Hematoma and distraction arthroplasty for basal thumb osteoarthritis. Tech Hand Up Extrem Surg 2004;8:2–6.

[39] Trumble TE, Rafijah G, Gilbert M, et al. Thumb trapeziometacarpal joint arthritis: partial trapeziectomy with ligament reconstruction and interposition costochondral allograft. J Hand Surg [Am] 2000;25:61–76.

[40] Nilsson A, Liljensten E, Bergstrom C, et al. Results from a degradable TMC joint spacer (Artelon) compared with tendon arthroplasty. J Hand Surg [Am] 2005;30:380–9.

[41] Badia A, Sambandam SN. Total joint arthroplasty in the treatment of advanced stages of thumb carpometacarpal joint osteoarthritis. J Hand Surg [Am] 2006;31:1605–14.

[42] Cooney WP, Linscheid RL, Askew LJ. Total arthroplasty of the thumb trapeziometacarpal joint. Clin Orthop Relat Res 1987;220:35–45.

[43] Moutet F, Lignon J, Oberlin C, et al. [Total trapeziometacarpal prostheses: results of a multicenter study (106 cases)]. Ann Chir Main Memb Super 1990;9:189–94 [in French].

[44] Gervis WH. Excision of the trapezium for osteoarthritis of the trapezio-metacarpal joint. J Bone Joint Surg Br 1949;31:537–9 [illust].

[45] Gray KV, Meals RA. Hematoma and distraction arthroplasty for thumb basal joint osteoarthritis: minimum 6.5-year follow-up evaluation. J Hand Surg [Am] 2007;32:23–9.

[46] Wajon A, Ada L, Edmunds I. Surgery for thumb (trapeziometacarpal joint) osteoarthritis. Cochrane Database Syst Rev 2005;4:CD004631.

[47] Wilson JN. Basal osteotomy of the first metacarpal in the treatment of arthritis of the carpometacarpal joint of the thumb. Br J Surg 1973;60:854–8.

[48] Hobby JL, Lyall HA, Meggitt BF. First metacarpal osteotomy for trapeziometacarpal osteoarthritis. J Bone Joint Surg Br 1998;80:508–12.

[49] Pellegrini VD Jr, Olcott CW, Hollenberg G. Contact patterns in the trapeziometacarpal joint: the role of the palmar beak ligament. J Hand Surg [Am] 1993; 18:238–44.

[50] Culp RW, Rekant MS. The role of arthroscopy in evaluating and treating trapeziometacarpal disease. Hand Clin 2001;17:315–9.

[51] Gonzalez MH, Kemmler J, Weinzweig N, et al. Portals for arthroscopy of the trapeziometacarpal joint. J Hand Surg [Br] 1997;22:574–5.

[52] Walsh EF, Akelman E, Fleming BC, et al. Thumb carpometacarpal arthroscopy: a topographic, anatomic study of the thenar portal. J Hand Surg [Am] 2005;30:373–9.

[53] Menon J. Arthroscopic management of trapeziometacarpal joint arthritis of the thumb. Arthroscopy 1996;12:581–7.

ELSEVIER
SAUNDERS

Hand Clin 24 (2008) 263–269

HAND
CLINICS

Treatment of Advanced Carpometacarpal Joint Disease: Carpometacarpal Arthroplasty with Ligament Interposition

Damien I. Davis, MD[a], Louis Catalano III, MD[b,c],*

[a]St. Luke's–Roosevelt Hospital Center, 1000 Tenth Avenue, New York, NY 10019, USA
[b]Columbia College of Physicians and Surgeons, 630 West 168th Street, New York, NY 10032, USA
[c]CV Starr Hand Surgery Center, St. Luke's–Roosevelt Hospital Center, 1000 Tenth Avenue 3rd Floor,
New York, NY 10019, USA

Basal joint arthritis is a common condition, primarily affecting postmenopausal women. Persistent pain and functional impairment despite conservative treatment are indications for operative intervention. Ligament reconstruction and tendon interposition (LRTI) arthroplasty is one of the most popular and time-tested operations to treat metacarpal instability and basal joint arthritis. LRTI incorporates three fundamental principles that address the underlying anatomic pathology: (1) trapezium excision, either partial or complete, to eliminate eburnated bone and the source of pain; (2) anterior oblique ligament reconstruction for carpometacarpal joint stability; and (3) tendon interposition to minimize axial shortening and prevent bony impingement. However, multiple procedures address these principles and discussion goes on as to which operation provides the most reliable outcomes.

Pathophysiology

Although there is an association between basal joint laxity and the subsequent development of arthritic changes, there is not complete agreement on which ligament is primarily responsible for maintaining joint stability. With compression forces as high as 120 kg measured at the

carpometacarpal joint during strong pinch, ligament integrity is thought to be essential in preventing translation of the metacarpal on the trapezium during thumb flexion [1].

There are four primary ligamentous constraints at the carpometacarpal joint of the thumb: (1) the anterior oblique ligament, (2) the dorsoradial ligament, (3) the posterior oblique ligament, and (4) the intermetacarpal ligament. Studies support each ligament as the primary stabilizer. The intermetacarpal ligament, which originates on the dorsoradial aspect of the index metacarpal and inserts onto the ulnar aspect of the first metacarpal base, was determined to be the primary restraint to dorsal and radial subluxation in a study by Pagalidis and colleagues [2]. The posterior oblique ligament, which originates on the dorsoulnar aspect of the trapezium and inserts on the palmar-ulnar tubercle of the first metacarpal base, was the principle stabilizer, according to Harvey and Bye [3]. Strauch and colleagues [4] performed serial sectioning of the ligaments of the carpometacarpal joint and showed that the primary restraint to dorsal dislocation was the dorsoradial ligament that connects the dorsal and radial aspect of the trapezium to the dorsum of the metacarpal base. Eaton [5,6] reported that the anterior oblique, or volar beak ligament, which originates on the palmar tubercle of the trapezium and inserts on the palmar ulnar tubercle at the base of the first metacarpal, is the primary restraint to dorsoradial subluxation. This theory is supported by anatomic studies showing a direct correlation between the degeneration of the

* Corresponding author. CV Starr Hand Surgery Center, St. Luke's–Roosevelt Hospital Center, 1000 Tenth Avenue 3rd Floor, New York, NY 10019.
  E-mail address: louiscatalano@msn.com (L. Catalano III).

trapeziometacarpal articular surface and the integrity of the beak ligament, as well as the clinical success of reconstructive basal joint surgery that recreates the functional anatomy of the beak ligament.

Pellegrini [1] performed a cadaver study that showed the beak ligament was the primary stabilizer of the thumb in pronation, while the dorsoradial ligament was the main stabilizer in the functionally less important position of supination. More importantly, he showed a significant difference between these two structures and their role in the development of degeneration of the articular cartilage of the trapeziometacarpal joint. Intact capsuloligamentous structures around the joint correlated with the presence of normal articular surfaces. Chondromalacia was observed in two distinct patterns: (1) localized in the dorsal compartment corresponding to the noncontact area during lateral pinch and (2) localized to the palmar compartment. In all instances of palmar chondromalacia, the beak ligament demonstrated degenerative changes. Eburnated bone only occurred in the palmar compartment and the area of eburnation corresponds to the primary loading area of the metacarpal and trapezium during lateral pinch. Trapeziometacarpal joints with eburnated bone all possessed degenerated beak ligaments, some displaying frank detachment of the ligament from the metacarpal insertion. In contrast, there was no correlation between the competency of the dorsoradial ligament and the degree of joint degeneration. Pellegrini concluded that the degeneration and incompetence of the anterior oblique ligament result in increased joint laxity and dorsal translation of the metacarpal on the trapezium when the thumb is in the position of lateral pinch. These pathologic processes cause increasing shear at the palmar compartment of the joint and the development of articular degeneration, resulting in possible eburnation. The major role the beak ligament plays in stabilizing the trapeziometacarpal joint, especially in the pronated position, is the reason its reconstruction is the focus of many procedures designed to reestablish thumb stability in cases of early- and late-stage osteoarthritis.

Evolution of procedures

Operative indications for basal joint arthritis include pain and weakness during activities of daily living in a compliant patient who has failed nonoperative treatment. The goals of surgery are to relieve pain and restore stability to the joint. Surgical options have evolved considerably since 1949 when Gervis first described trapezium excision for osteoarthritis of the trapeziometacarpal joint. Over the past 58 years, myriad procedures have been developed. While the biomechanical principles of many of these surgeries are similar, there is still controversy as to which of the various procedures provides the best long-term outcomes. The choice of procedure depends on the individual pathology of the patient. The key anatomic findings that determine the necessary operation are the presence or absence of degeneration at the scaphotrapezial joint, as well as hyperextension at the metacarpophalangeal joint.

LRTI arthroplasty is one of the most popular and time-tested operations to treat metacarpal instability and basal joint arthritis. This procedure incorporates three fundamental principles that address the underlying anatomic pathology: (1) trapezium excision, either partial or complete, to eliminate eburnated bone and the source of pain, (2) anterior oblique ligament reconstruction for carpometacarpal joint stability, and (3) tendon interposition to minimize axial shortening and prevent bony impingement.

Results

LRTI is an amalgamation of procedures, each of which corrected one of the previously mentioned principles of basal joint surgery. Trapezium excision was first described in 1949 by Gervis [7], who subsequently had his own trapezium excised in 1971 [8]. The long-term results of this operation were satisfactory but concern arose regarding loss of thumb length and decreased pinch strength. A variation of trapezium excision, termed hematoma-distraction arthroplasty, has gained renewed interest. This procedure augments Gervis' trapezium excision with fixation of the thumb metacarpal to the index metacarpal in a distracted position via Kirschner wires. Four to 5 weeks of the thumb pinned in distraction is intended to promote scarring and fibrous tissue formation in the area of the excised trapezium and decrease axial shortening, which was thought to contribute to poor outcomes seen with traditional excision. Gray and Meals [9] prospectively followed 22 thumbs that were treated via hematoma-distraction arthroplasty with trapeziectomy and 5 weeks of Kirschner-wire immobilization with the metacarpal in opposition and distraction. At follow-up at a mean of 88 months, 18 out of

22 patients were pain-free. Strength measurements showed an average of 21% increase in grip strength and tip-pinch strength, and an 11% increase in key-pinch strength. While investigators reported metacarpal subsidence, they found no correlation with subjective or objective outcomes.

In 1970, Froimson [10] described tendon interposition in addition to trapezium excision to address metacarpal subsidence and decreased pinch strength. His residents termed the procedure the "anchovy operation" because of the similar appearance of the rolled tendon graft and the food. He reported universal relief of pain in his series of 80 procedures in 72 patients. However, long-term follow-up still showed reduced pinch strength, as well as axial shortening. Pinch power was consistently reduced by 30% and radiographic measurement demonstrated 50% decrease in space between the base of the first metacarpal and scaphoid, which resulted in negligible thumb shortening [11].

The third treatment principle is restoration of metacarpal stability by volar ligament reconstruction and was first described by Eaton and Littler in 1973. This procedure is indicated for stage I disease, with the joint surfaces demonstrating minimal chondromalacia at the palmar compartment of the trapeziometacarpal joint. More advanced articular degeneration at the trapeziometacarpal joint or scaphotrapezial joint involvement precludes the use of this operation as the sole treatment. Eaton and Littler [5] reported the results of 18 patients with minimum follow-up of 1 year and noted a direct correlation between outcomes and degree of articular degeneration. They reported 11 excellent, 5 good, and 2 fair outcomes. Of the 11 patients with excellent results, 3 were in stage I preoperatively, 2 were stage II, 5 were stage III, and 1 was stage IV. Of the 5 with good results, the disease in 3 preoperatively was classified as stage III and in 2 as stage IV. The 2 patients with fair results were both stage IV preoperatively.

Originally described by Burton and Pellegrini in 1986, ligament reconstruction with tendon interposition encompasses all of the treatment principles that were previously addressed individually by Gervis, Froimson, and Eaton and Littler. Burton and Pellegrini [12] reported excellent results in 92% of cases (23 out of 25 thumbs). Their version of the LRTI involved harvesting half of the flexor carpi radialis (FCR) tendon and excising either the distal half of the trapezium (6 cases) or removing the entire trapezium (19 cases) if degenerative changes were observed in the scaphotrapezial joint. Grip and pinch strength increased 19% compared with preoperative values. Radiographically, there was an average decrease of 11% of the immediate postoperative arthroplasty space secondary to metacarpal subsidence. In 1995, Tomaino and colleagues [13] performed a long-term follow-up, averaging 9 years, of Burton and Pellegrini's original patients. The average grip strength at 9-year follow-up demonstrated an improvement of 93% compared with preoperative values. The average tip-pinch strength improved 65% and key-pinch improved 34% compared with preoperative levels. Loss of height of the arthroplasty space averaged 13% on stress radiographs at 9 years postoperatively. They concluded that thumb function continues to improve for up to 6 years following LRTI and that the procedure is both reliable and durable.

De Smet and colleagues [14] challenged the notion that thumb subsidence associated with simple trapeziectomy was responsible for reduced grip and key-pinch strength. They analyzed two cohorts: one group, consisting of 22 patients, undergoing trapeziectomy, and the other, 34 patients, receiving LRTI with mean follow-up of 26 to 34 months. The investigators then compared subjective and objective criteria. Trapezial space was better maintained in the LRTI group with a loss of height of 32% compared with preoperative level versus 57.5% height decrease in the trapeziectomy group. However, their results showed no statistically significant differences for pain relief, patient satisfaction, Disabilities of the Arm, Shoulder and Hand (DASH) score, key-pinch force, or gripping force, although it did show a correlation between maintenance of thumb height and key-pinch force.

In a prospective, randomized study, Kriegs-Au and colleagues [15] compared trapezial excision with ligament reconstruction alone (group I) to trapezium excision with ligament reconstruction combined with tendon interposition (group II). Mean follow-up was 48.2 months and no significant differences could be detected between the groups for tip-pinch or grip strength. In addition the data showed no statistically significant difference between the two groups with regard to height of the arthroplasty space. Group I demonstrated a 42% average height loss at 4 years compared with immediate postoperative arthroplasty space and group II displayed a 37% loss of height. Regression analyses showed no significant relationship between tip-pinch strength and the decrease in height of the arthroplasty space. Krieg-Au and colleagues concluded that tendon interposition does not affect the outcomes of ligament reconstruction and metacarpal subsidence may have no effect on postoperative thumb strength, function, and pain.

This was supported by Lins and colleagues [16], who performed a retrospective study of 30 thumbs that underwent LRTI. Their results showed a 50% increase in grip strength and 43% increase in pinch strength with a mean follow-up of 42 months, which are similar to long-term results obtained by Tomaino and colleagues. They also measured trapezial space ratio, which is the space defined by the distal scaphoid and thumb metacarpal base divided by the thumb proximal phalanx on radiograph. Lins and colleagues reported a decrease in this ratio of 33% from before surgery to after LRTI, but noted no significant correlation between this decrease and patient satisfaction, grip and pinch strengths, and ability to return to activities of daily living.

Procedure

The procedure begins with the patient in a supine position with a tourniquet secured around the arm. The incision is centered over the dorsal aspect of the trapeziometacarpal joint. The authors use a longitudinal dorsal incision at the glabrous-nonglabrous skin interval (Fig. 1). Following the skin incision, meticulous dissection of the subcutaneous tissues is required to protect the superficial branches of the radial sensory nerve and the radial artery (Fig. 2).

To expose the joint, a longitudinal capsular incision is made. This incision should be extended

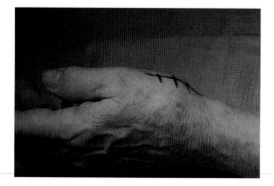

Fig. 1. Longitudinal skin incision at glabrous-nonglabrous interface.

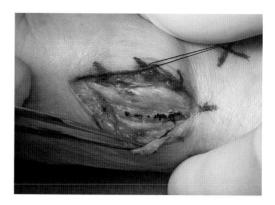

Fig. 2. Superficial branch of radial sensory nerve protected by forceps.

proximally enough so that the scaphotrapezial joint can be visualized. To gain access to the capsule, the extensor pollicus longus is retracted in a dorsal and ulnar direction while the abductor pollicus longus is retracted radially and volarly. The trapezium can be excised either en masse or in fragments. Removing the trapezium in fragments requires it to be cut into quadrants by bisecting it both longitudinally and transversely with a sagittal saw or osteotome. Care must be taken not to penetrate the far cortex of the trapezium with the saw or osteotome as the FCR runs along the palmar crest of the trapezium. The next step requires preparation of the thumb metacarpal. The base of the metacarpal, including the entire articular surface, is cut using a saw perpendicular to its long axis. A bone tunnel is made with the use of a 3-mm burr or a similar-sized gouge. The tunnel should start along the metacarpal shaft approximately 1 cm distal to the base and perpendicular to the thumbnail plate. The other end of the tunnel should exit at the volar beak of the metacarpal base. This allows the course of the harvested FCR tendon to anatomically reapproximate the insertion of the volar beak ligament.

The FCR tendon is harvested via a 1.5-cm transverse incision in the volar forearm at the musculotendinous junction. In Burton and Pellegrini's [12] original description of the procedure in 1986, he advocated harvesting only the radial half of the tendon. He later modified the procedure to include harvesting the entire FCR tendon. The authors also use the entire FCR tendon (Fig. 3). Tomaino and Coleman [17] showed there was no significant morbidity regarding wrist strength or endurance when harvesting the entire FCR tendon. When harvesting half of the FCR tendon,

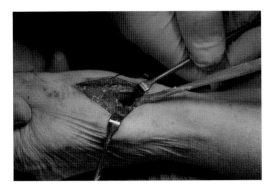

Fig. 3. Trapezium excised and harvested FCR tendon brought through incision in preparation for interposition.

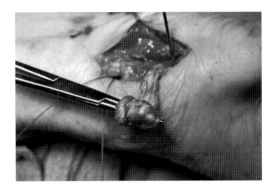

Fig. 4. FCR tendon rolled onto itself to form the "anchovy".

note that proximally, the ulnar half should be divided and passed distally. There is a 180° axial rotation of the tendon as it courses distally, resulting in the proximal, ulnar half becoming the distal, radial half of the tendon. The distal, radial half of the tendon is in a better anatomic position for ligament reconstruction [18].

The free end of the harvested tendon is tapered to allow it to pass easily through the metacarpal bone tunnel. The volar capsule of the joint is easily visualized and prepared with two Vicryl sutures for subsequent stabilization of the tendon "anchovy" once the graft is tensioned. Metacarpal stabilization and tendon tensioning are two of the key aspects of the procedure. Proper tensioning of the FCR graft helps prevent proximal migration and radial subluxation of the thumb [12]. Longitudinal traction is applied to the thumb to maintain the space from which the trapezium was excised. The base of the thumb metacarpal should be at the level of the index carpometacarpal joint. The orientation of the thumb should be in the key-pinch position, which is extension-abduction. A 0.045-in diameter (or 0.054-in diameter in larger hands) Kirschner wire is inserted obliquely from the dorsoradial aspect of the thumb metacarpal into the base of the index metacarpal. The free end of the FCR tendon is then passed through the base of the thumb metacarpal and out of the hole at the dorsoradial aspect of the shaft. The tendon is subsequently tensioned and sutured to the lateral periosteum of the metacarpal and then back to itself to resurface at the base of the metacarpal [12]. The remaining tendon is folded over onto itself several times to form the "anchovy," which is secured with sutures in each corner (Fig. 4). The two previously placed sutures in the volar capsule are

then passed from volar to dorsal through the anchovy and the graft is dropped down to occupy the arthroplasty space, becoming the tendon interposition (Fig. 5). Fig. 6 shows a radiograph after LRTI with a suture anchor in the trapezoid, which is the authors' preferred way to anchor the tendon graft in the arthroplasty space. The capsule is closed over the anchovy, taking care to protect the superficial branches of the radial sensory nerve and the radial artery. The patient is placed in a short-arm thumb-spica splint for the immediate postoperative period.

Once the basal joint reconstruction is complete, attention must be focused on the thumb metacarpophalangeal joint. It is important to note preoperatively if there is any evidence of thumb metacarpophalangeal hyperextensibility. Conventional teaching supports the idea that

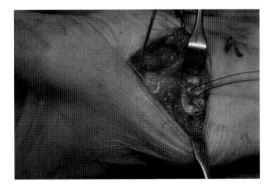

Fig. 5. The two previously placed sutures in the volar capsule are seen, having been passed from volar to dorsal through the anchovy and the graft has been dropped down to occupy the arthroplasty space, becoming the tendon interposition. The Kirschner wire, seen at the proximal aspect of the incision, stabilizes the thumb metacarpal to the index metacarpal.

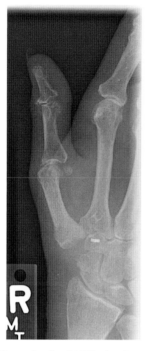

Fig. 6. Radiograph after LRTI, showing arthroplasty space and suture anchor in trapezoid to secure tendon interposition.

instability that develops at the metacarpophalangeal joint is compensatory in response to subluxation at the trapeziometacarpal joint. Moulton and colleagues [19] believe that in some patients the increased laxity of the metacarpophalangeal joint contributes to, rather than results from, trapeziometacarpal joint degeneration. Hyperextension at the thumb metacarpophalangeal joint causes increased metacarpal flexion and adduction, especially during lateral pinch. These augmented vectors may result in metacarpophalangeal joint collapse, placing increased stress on ligament reconstruction and the carpometacarpal joint, possibly leading to poor surgical outcomes. Burton and Pellegrini describe routinely transferring the extensor pollicus brevis tendon from its insertion on the base of the proximal phalanx of the thumb to the metacarpal shaft to remove a hyperextension force at the metacarpophalangeal joint and enhance the metacarpal abduction vector. Treatment of the metacarpophalangeal joint is dependent on the degree of hyperextension. If the hyperextension is less than 20° to 30°, treatment options include observation or placement of a Kirschner wire obliquely across

the metacarpophalangeal joint to hold it in flexion for 6 weeks. If hyperextension is greater than 30°, treatment options include arthrodesis in 5° to 10° of flexion or volar capsulodesis. By securing the metacarpophalangeal joint in flexion, the more severely involved palmar compartment of the trapeziometacarpal joint is unloaded, resulting in a shift of the contact pressure toward the dorsal compartment [19]. A grossly unstable or degenerative metacarpophalangeal joint is more amenable to arthrodesis.

Postoperative care

The choice of postoperative therapy regimens depends upon both the protocol of the surgeon and the preoperative functional status of the patient. Older, lower-demand patients may not require extensive postoperative hand therapy. Suture removal occurs on postoperative day 10 with application of a thumb spica cast. Immobilization continues in a thumb spica cast for 6 weeks, at which time the Kirschner wires are removed. After 6 weeks of casting, the patient is transitioned into a removable thumb spica splint. Gentle wrist and thumb metacarpophalangeal joint range-of-motion exercises may be initiated at this time. Metacarpal abduction and extension are begun first, followed by flexion-adduction and opposition, which are not emphasized until week 8. At 6 weeks, thenar isometric strengthening may be initiated, followed by pinch and grip strengthening at 8 weeks. Splinting is continued during this postoperative period until range of motion and strength are restored, which most often is achieved by 12 weeks. Patients should be informed that range of motion, grip strength, and pinch strength can all continue to improve for up to 1 year after surgery.

Summary

There are numerous surgical procedures for basal joint arthritis. In addition to correcting carpometacarpal joint pathology, the metacarpophalangeal joint must also be addressed at the time of surgery, regardless of which operation is performed. The authors' preferred treatment is ligament reconstruction and tendon interposition. The components of reliable surgical outcomes include trapeziectomy, ligament reconstruction, and tendon interposition. Many studies based on long-term follow-up support trapeziectomy alone [9,14,20], trapeziectomy plus ligament reconstruction without tendon interposition [15], and trapeziectomy plus ligament reconstruction with tendon interposition [12,13]. Basal joint arthritis is a common problem that may be treated via various reconstructive procedures reliably resulting in decreased pain and high patient satisfaction rates.

References

[1] Pellegrini VD. Osteoarthritis of the trapeziometacarpal joint: the pathophysiology of articular cartilage degeneration. I. Anatomy and pathology of the aging joint. J Hand Surg [Am] 1991;16A: 967–74.

[2] Pagalidis T, Kuczynski K, Lamb DW. Ligamentous stability of the base of the thumb. Hand 1981;13: 29–35.

[3] Harvey FJ, Bye WD. Bennett's fracture. Hand 1976; 8:48–53.

[4] Strauch RJ, Behrman MJ, Rosenwasser MP. Acute dislocation of the carpometacarpal joint of the thumb: an anatomic and cadaver study. J Hand Surg [Am] 1994;19A:93–8.

[5] Eaton RG, Littler JW. Ligament reconstruction for the painful thumb carpometacarpal joint. J Bone Joint Surg Am 1973;55:1655–66.

[6] Eaton RG, Glickel SZ. Trapeziometacarpal osteoarthritis: staging as a rationale for treatment. Hand Clin 1987;3:455–71.

[7] Gervis WH. Excision of the trapezium for osteoarthritis of the trapeziometacarpal joint. J Bone Joint Surg Br 1949;31:537–9.

[8] Gervis WH. A review of excision of the trapezium for osteoarthritis of the trapezio-metacarpal joint after twenty-five years. J Bone Joint Surg Br 1973; 55B:56–7.

[9] Gray KV, Meals RA. Hematoma and distraction arthroplasty for thumb basal joint osteoarthritis: minimum 6.5-year follow-up evaluation. J Hand Surg [Am] 2007;32:23–9.

[10] Froimson AI. Tendon arthroplasty of the trapeziometacarpal joint. Clin Orthop 1970;70:191–9.

[11] Froimson AI. Tendon interposition arthroplasty of carpometacarpal joint of the thumb. Hand Clin 1987;3:489–505.

[12] Burton RI, Pellegrini VD. Surgical management of basal joint arthritis of the thumb. Part II. Ligament reconstruction with tendon interposition arthroplasty. J Hand Surg [Am] 1986;11A:324–32.

[13] Tomaino MM, Pellegrini VD, Burton RI. Arthroplasty of the basal joint of the thumb. Long-term follow-up after ligament reconstruction with tendon interposition. J Bone Joint Surg Am 1995;77:346–55.

[14] De Smet L, Sioen W, Spaepen D, et al. Treatment of basal joint arthritis of the thumb: trapeziectomy with or without tendon interposition/ligament reconstruction. Hand Surg 2004;9:5–9.

[15] Kriegs-Au G, Petje G, Fotjl E, et al. Ligament reconstruction with or without tendon interposition to treat primary thumb carpometacarpal osteoarthritis. A prospective randomized study. J Bone Joint Surg Am 2004;86:209–18.

[16] Lins RE, Gelberman RH, McKeown L, et al. Basal joint arthritis: trapeziectomy with ligament reconstruction and tendon interposition arthroplasty. J Hand Surg [Am] 1996;21A:202–9.

[17] Tomaino MM, Coleman K. Use of the entire width of the flexor carpi radialis tendon for the LRTI arthroplasty does not impair wrist function. Am J Orthop 2000;29:283–4.

[18] Barron OA, Glickel SZ, Eaton RG. Basal joint arthritis of the thumb. J Am Acad Orthop Surg 2000;8:314–23.

[19] Moulton MJR, Parentis MA, Kelly MJ, et al. Influence of metacarpophalangeal joint position on basal joint-loading in the thumb. J Bone Joint Surg Am 2001;83A:709–16.

[20] Kuhns CA, Emerson ET, Meals RA. Hematomadistraction arthroplasty for thumb basal joint osteoarthritis: a prospective, single-surgeon study including outcomes measures. J Hand Surg [Am] 2003;28(3):381–9.

ELSEVIER
SAUNDERS

Hand Clin 24 (2008) 271–276

HAND
CLINICS

Treatment of Advanced Carpometacarpal Joint Disease: Trapeziectomy and Hematoma Arthroplasty

Brian T. Fitzgerald, MD*, Eric P. Hofmeister, MD

*Division of Hand and Microvascular Surgery, Department of Orthopaedic Surgery,
Naval Medical Center San Diego, 34800 Bob Wilson Drive, Suite 112, San Diego, CA 92131, USA*

Osteoarthritis of the thumb basal joint is a common entity affecting primarily postmenopausal women. Symptoms of pain and eventual difficulty with dexterity and grasping can significantly debilitate patients. Diagnosis can be made with a history, physical examination, and radiographic evaluation. Radiographs may show less impressive evidence of degenerative changes than would be expected based on subjective complaints; however, there can be advanced arthritic changes that are confirmatory of the disease (Fig. 1). When the most common first-line treatments, such as rest, splinting, medications, and steroid injections, no longer adequately alleviate pain, surgical options are appropriate to consider.

The primary goal of surgical treatment of the osteoarthritic first trapeziometacarpal (TM) joint is pain relief. The preservation of functional range of motion and adequate strength and stability are important secondary objectives. There continues to be controversy among surgeons who treat significantly painful basal joint arthritis as to the ideal operative procedure to offer patients. Because many methods of surgical treatment exist and continue to be used, it can be inferred that no one procedure is clearly superior to another.

Simple trapezial excision without soft tissue interposition was first described by Gervis [1] in 1949. Many other reports have since been published on this procedure [2–18]. Unsatisfactory results with the procedure during the 1950s and the ensuing two decades ultimately led to the development of more complex arthroplasty options and suspensionplasty procedures [19–21]. In the past 5 to 10 years, interest in the use of simple trapeziectomy with modifications to the original description has been renewed.

Many authorities agree that there is a high likelihood of significant pain relief with trapeziectomy. The often-cited drawbacks of the procedure have included loss of thumb strength and stability [2,5,19,22]. In one report, the loss of power grip that was noted from the procedure was described as "an acceptable price to pay" for pain relief [2]. Although grip and pinch strength are often decreased after surgery, the absence or marked decrease in pain results in improved overall function and reasonable functional grip. Supporters of this procedure argue that, although strength is not returned to normal, it is improved in most patients. Much of the current literature focuses on the clinical significance of any loss of height of the arthroplasty space, altered joint kinematics of the thumb, grip and pinch strength, and range of motion that may or may not support the continued use of this treatment option for advanced TM arthritis.

Based on the simplicity and low morbidity of the procedure, as well as multiple reports on the success rates that compare well with other techniques of carpometacarpal (CMC)

The views expressed in this article are those of the authors and do not reflect the official policy or position of the Department of the Navy, Department of Defense, or the United States Government.

* Corresponding author.

E-mail address: brian.fitzgerald@med.navy.mil (B.T. Fitzgerald).

0749-0712/08/$ - see front matter. Published by Elsevier Inc.
doi:10.1016/j.hcl.2008.03.003

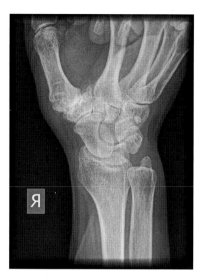

Fig. 1. Radiograph of a patient with advanced CMC arthritis of the thumb.

arthroplasty, trapeziectomy with hematoma arthroplasty has been increasingly used in clinical practice.

Indications

Elective surgery to address pain resulting from CMC arthritis is reasonable to offer patients when nonoperative measures no longer alleviate symptoms to a functional level or when the patient feels he or she is significantly limited by pain. Some authorities have advocated simple trapeziectomy with hematoma arthroplasty only for salvage situations, such as after a failed or infected implant arthroplasty [22,23]. In 2000, the opinion of prominent authorities was that trapezium excision should be limited to low-demand, elderly patients without significant metacarpal base subluxation [24]. Nevertheless, the authors agree with previously described indications [25] and believe it is a clinically proven option as a primary treatment and recommend it to patients who have significantly limiting pain. Patient selection and realistic patient expectations are critical to a successful outcome. An exception to performing this procedure would be a young active patient who requires preservation of strenuous grasp and pinch strength for work or activities of daily living. These patients are better served by a well-performed metacarpal osteotomy or fusion depending on the degree of joint involvement.

Surgical technique

Trapeziectomy can be performed under regional block or general anesthesia and with tourniquet control. Other procedures as needed should be performed in the same setting, such as carpal tunnel release, first extensor compartment release, or metacarpal-phalangeal stabilization. A single dose of perioperative antibiotics is given (cefazolin or clindamycin) before incision.

A longitudinal incision is made along the glabrous margin of the skin on the radial border of the thumb metacarpal, just volar to the course of the extensor pollicis brevis (EPB) tendon. The incision is centered over the trapezium, approximately 1 cm proximal to the thumb metacarpal base. Sharp dissection is carried through the skin, and blunt dissection is made through the subcutaneous tissues. Care is taken to identify and protect branches of the dorsal sensory radial nerve. It is beneficial to keep these nerve branches within the perineural fat and moist throughout the case. The EPB and abductor pollicis longus (APL) tendons are identified. The interval between these tendons is deepened. Alternatively, the EPB tendon can be retracted volarly along with the APL and dissection to the joint capsule continued dorsal to both tendons. The radial artery should be identified coursing through the surgical field at the level of the scaphotrapezial joint, superficial to the capsule. Any branch of the artery found entering the capsule over the trapezium can be cauterized.

Once the joint capsule is exposed, it is opened longitudinally, and volar and dorsal flaps are developed sharply. It is helpful to tag these flaps with suture for later identification during closure. The flaps are developed from 0.5 cm distal to the base of the metacarpal, proximally to the level of the scaphotrapezial joint. Removal of the trapezium is greatly facilitated by maximal reflection of the capsule from all accessible attachments to the bone. A freer elevator or blunt probe is inserted into the presumed TM joint, and a fluoroscopic image is taken to confirm the location. A cruciate osteotomy is made in the trapezium with a small osteotome or oscillating saw blade. Penetration through the full thickness of bone is not advised with a saw blade, because the flexor carpi radialis (FCR) tendon courses deep to the dorsal trapezial cortex and may be inadvertently injured. The fractionation of the trapezium is completed with an osteotome, and piecemeal removal is performed with rongeurs. Visual inspection to confirm the integrity of the FCR tendon is made, and fluoroscopic imaging is used to ensure complete bony excision and removal of all osteophytes. The authors routinely inspect the scaphotrapezoidal joint as well; partial excision of the trapezoid can be performed if significant arthritis is present.

Following complete removal of all bone fragments from the arthroplasty space, the thumb metacarpal is stabilized with a minimum of one percutaneous 0.062-in K-wire (Fig. 2). This stabilization is done by positioning the thumb metacarpal base at the same level as the index finger metacarpal base via longitudinal traction, with 2 mm of joint space between the two. Slight pronation and wide palmar abduction are maintained, and the pins are placed from the thumb metacarpal base into the index metacarpal. Alternatively, the pins can be advanced from the thumb metacarpal into the trapezoid. Rigid fixation is confirmed, and correct pin positioning is documented by fluoroscopy. To ensure adequate thumb abduction and pronation, a fist is passively formed, noting the location of the thumb tip. Ideally, this should overlay the middle and ring fingers distal to the proximal interphalangeal joints. Pins are left protruding through the skin.

The joint capsule, previously tagged with suture, is closed with 3-0 or 4-0 absorbable suture. Hemostasis is evaluated by releasing the tourniquet and assessing for any arterial bleeding. The skin is closed with absorbable sutures. The metacarpophalangeal joint is examined, and any significant hyperextension is addressed. A forearm-based thumb spica splint is applied. The patient is seen 7 to 10 days postoperatively and placed into a short arm, thumb spica cast with the interphalangeal joint left free. The cast and pins are removed 5 weeks after surgery, and formal hand therapy is initiated with active motion exercises and continued support of the thumb with a removable thumb spica splint for the next 2 to 3 weeks. Extreme movements of the thumb are avoided for approximately 3 months after surgery, and, at this point, no limitations are imposed on patients (Fig. 3).

Results after trapezial excision alone

Despite poor results of trapeziectomy and hematoma arthroplasty in treating first CMC arthritis in the 1950s, a newfound interest regarding this technique is found in the literature. Multiple retrospective reviews have demonstrated the clinical success of simple trapezial excision. Dhar and colleagues [6] reported that excellent pain relief and "reasonable strength" and motion were obtained at an average follow-up of 6 years. They found no statistically significant grip or pinch strength differences, but did note that maximal function was not obtained for approximately 9 months. A reduction of pinch strength but greater than 75% rate of pain relief at a median

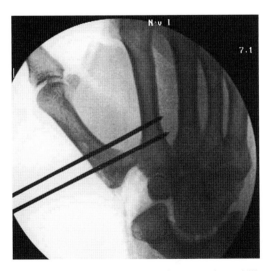

Fig. 2. Intraoperative fluoroscopy demonstrating stabilization of the thumb metacarpal to the index metacarpal in a slightly overdistracted position.

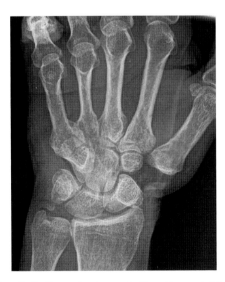

Fig. 3. Radiograph demonstrating the maintained arthroplasty space after removal of pins in a patient 3 months postoperative.

5-year follow-up was demonstrated by Varley and colleagues [7]. Hollovoet and colleagues [8] found no statistically significant difference in motion, strength, or trapezial space height between simple trapeziectomy and soft tissue interpositional arthroplasty. Vandenbroucke and colleagues [10] found that pinch strength was consistently diminished when compared with preoperative values, but 85% of patients were pain free at 2 years. The conclusions of Belcher were that ligament reconstruction and tendon interposition (LRTI) conferred no additional benefit to trapezial excision based on a randomized case series, although follow-up averaged only 13 months [12]. The common technique factor among these case series is that all of the patients were either mobilized early or immobilized for no more than 3 to 4 weeks but not pinned in a distracted position.

More recently, renewed interest has led to modifications that include keeping the thumb distracted and immobilized for several weeks after surgery, allowing a hematoma to organize in the arthroplasty space and the remaining capsular structures to consolidate sufficiently enough to secure the metacarpal base. In a prospective study of 13 patients, the trapezial gap was measured preoperatively and at 2, 4, and 12 weeks after undergoing a trapeziectomy without pinning of the first metacarpal [26]. Collapse of this space was noted up to 4 weeks postoperatively; no further collapse followed this time frame, despite the cessation of splinting. This observation implies there is utility to leaving a stabilizing pin in place for a minimum of 4 weeks postoperatively.

A prospective study of 69 thumbs comparing trapeziectomy alone, trapeziectomy with palmaris longus tendon interposition, or trapeziectomy with LRTI involved uniformly pinning the first metacarpal to the distal pole of the scaphoid, regardless of which procedure was performed [13]. The goal was to prevent migration of the first metacarpal and to determine which method was more effective in maintaining trapezial space height. At 1 year follow-up, no statistically significant decrease was seen in the trapezial space ratios in the three treatment groups, and no significant difference of thumb key and pinch strengths was seen among the groups. Also, the researchers found no significant positive correlation between preservation of the trapezial space height and thumb strength at 1 year.

In a large study of 183 thumbs, these same three procedures were examined, again at 1 year follow-up [16]. As in the previous study, all three

groups had pinning of the first metacarpal for 4 weeks in addition to 6 weeks of immobilization. The results showed that 82% of the patients achieved good pain relief, 68% regained sufficient strength to allow resumption of activities of daily living, and key pinch significantly improved in all three groups, regardless of the surgery performed. There were no cases of subluxation or dislocations of the thumb. This well-performed study has provided evidence that the results of trapeziectomy alone are comparable with that of other arthroplasty options.

In a small prospective study of 56 thumbs comparing trapeziectomy without pinning with LRTI, no differences in pain relief, patient satisfaction, mobility, disabilities of the arm, shoulder and hand scores, key pinch strength, or grip strength were observed [15]; however, in contrast to the previous study, trapezial height was much better preserved in the LRTI group, and the remaining trapezial space did significantly correlate with key pinch force.

Kuhns and colleagues [14] in a prospective study of 26 thumbs from a single surgeon's practice reported on the results of trapezial excision and K-wire immobilization in a slightly overcorrected position for 5 weeks. At 6 months, 19 patients (73%) reported complete relief of pain, 24 could fully adduct thumb into the plane of their palm, and 25 could oppose their thumb to the fifth metacarpal head. At 24 months postoperatively, strength measurements showed an average 47% increase in grip strength, 33% increase in key pinch, and 23% increase in tip strength. It was theorized that the hematoma that develops in the arthroplasty space undergoes fibrosis with time and becomes organized into adequately supportive tissue for the thumb metacarpal.

A follow-up study in 2007 was reported by the same senior author (RAM) on this technique with the results at 6.5 years after operation [18]. Twenty-two thumb surgeries were reviewed, and 18 were entirely pain free. Twenty-one patients could fully abduct the thumb into the plane of their palm, and 21 could oppose their thumb to the fifth metacarpal head. Strength measurements had decreased from the previous publication but still showed an average 21% increase in grip strength and tip pinch strength, and 11% of patients demonstrated an increase in key pinch strength. These studies highlight that traziectomy without a formal ligament reconstruction allows for restoration and maintenance of a stable, pain-free thumb when compared with more complicated surgical interventions.

Discussion

Trapeziectomy with hematoma arthroplasty has continued to gain support as a reliable technique for treating painful CMC arthritis. Among its advantages are the straightforward nature of the procedure, reduced operative times, decreased anesthetic requirements, lack of need for expensive implants or allograft, and obviation of the need for donor tendon graft harvest.

Perhaps the reason results have improved since the 1950s lies in the fact that modifications have been popularized in recent years. Essential to the success of the operation is the development of a fibrous pseudarthrosis in the arthroplasty space from maturation of the postoperative hematoma. Additionally, the ligamentous support that remains after trapeziectomy helps maintain thumb metacarpal length [25]. Slightly overdistracting the first metacarpal relative to the index metacarpal likely enhances the ability of the thumb to heal with adequate stability [18].

Concerns over potential risks and disadvantages unique to the procedure continue to stimulate research and discussion, but a growing body of evidence supports that, given enough time and appropriate temporary fixation, the thumb will predictably become adequately stable, functionally mobile, and less painful. Because excision of the trapezium creates a loss of integrity of the scaphotrapezial-trapezoidal ligament, the initial concern was that carpal instability could result postoperatively; however, at greater than 3 years after surgery, Herren and colleagues [27] showed no evidence of carpal instability.

Concerns regarding the failure to maintain normal trapezial space height and the effects thereof have been studied. Even when performed with LRTI, this procedure may not be effective in restoring the arthroplasty space, but it gives "uniformly satisfactory clinical outcomes" [28]. Multiple other reports have concluded that no correlation exists between the amount of metacarpal subsidence and the clinical outcome after trapeziectomy [4,13,18]; therefore, to criticize trapeziectomy for allowing a similar loss of postoperative space height is of questionable validity.

The additional morbidity of tendon graft harvest, bone tunnel placement, and graft manipulation are all avoided with trapeziectomy and hematoma arthroplasty. This factor does not lessen the potential for other surgical risks, such as sensory radial nerve injury or radial arterial injury, which still must be minimized by careful technique and anatomic expertise. With any CMC arthroplasty procedure, metacarpophalangeal instability and adduction contracture should be evaluated. Despite one surgeon's experience that these secondary deformities spontaneous correct after trapeziectomy and hematoma arthroplasty [25], the authors believe they should still be evaluated intraoperatively and addressed.

Summary

Simple trapeziectomy is a clinically proven, effective technique with low morbidity that is useful in treating painful CMC arthritis. Support for this procedure has been demonstrated in multiple quality studies in the European and American literature. This body of knowledge, as well as the authors' experience, support that it is comparable to other arthroplasty methods, including formal LRTI. A longer-term prospective comparison of simple trapeziectomy with LRTI may determine whether the recent popularity of the former will be borne out by comparable or more favorable outcomes.

References

[1] Gervis WH. Excision of the trapezium for osteoarthritis of the trapezio-metacarpal joint. J Bone Joint Surg Br 1949;31:537–9.

[2] Murley AH. Excision of the trapezium in osteoarthritis of the first carpo-metacarpal joint. J Bone Joint Surg Br 1960;42:502–7.

[3] Gervis WH. A review of excision of the trapezium for osteoarthritis of the trapezio-metacarpal joint after twenty-five years. J Bone Joint Surg Br 1973; 55:56–7.

[4] Dell PC, Brushart TM, Smith RJ. Treatment of trapeziometacarpal arthritis: results of resection arthroplasty. J Hand Surg [Am] 1978;3:243–9.

[5] Iyer KM. The results of excision of the trapezium. Hand 1981;13:246–50.

[6] Dhar S, Gray IC, Jones WA, et al. Simple excision of the trapezium for osteoarthritis of the carpometacarpal joint of the thumb. J Hand Surg [Br] 1994; 19:485–8.

[7] Varley GW, Calvey J, Hunter JB, et al. Excision of the trapezium for osteoarthritis at the base of the thumb. J Bone Joint Surg Br 1994;76:964–8.

[8] Hollovoet N, Kinnen L, Moermans JP, et al. Excision of the trapezium for osteoarthritis of the trapeziometacarpal joint of the thumb. J Hand Surg [Br] 1996;21:458–62.

[9] Davis TR, Brady O, Barton NJ, et al. Trapeziectomy alone, with tendon interposition, or with ligament reconstruction? J Hand Surg [Br] 1997;22:689–94.

[10] Vandenbroucke J, DeSchriver F, DeSmet L, et al. Simple trapeziectomy for treatment of trapeziometacarpal osteoarthritis of the thumb. Clin Rheumatol 1997;16:239–42.

[11] Gibbons CE, Gosal HS, Choudri AH, et al. Trapeziectomy for basal thumb joint osteoarthritis: 3- to 19-year follow-up. Int Orthop 1999;23:216–8.

[12] Belcher HJ, Nicholl JE. A comparison of trapeziectomy with and without ligament reconstruction and tendon interposition. J Hand Surg [Br] 2000;25:350–6.

[13] Downing ND, Davis TR. Trapezial space height after trapeziectomy: mechanism of formation and benefits. J Hand Surg [Am] 2001;26:862–8.

[14] Kuhns CA, Emerson ET, Meals RA. Hematoma and distraction arthroplasty for thumb basal joint osteoarthritis: a prospective, single-surgeon study including outcomes measures. J Hand Surg [Am] 2003;28:381–9.

[15] DeSmet L, Sioen W, Spaepen D, et al. Treatment of basal joint arthritis of the thumb: trapeziectomy with or without tendon interposition/ligament reconstruction. Hand Surg 2004;9:5–9.

[16] Davis TR, Brady O, Dias JJ. Excision of the trapezium for osteoarthritis of the trapeziometacarpal joint: a study of the benefit of ligament reconstruction or tendon interposition. J Hand Surg [Am] 2004;29:1069–77.

[17] Mahoney JD, Meals RA. Trapeziectomy. Hand Clin 2006;22:165–9.

[18] Gray KV, Meals RA. Hematoma and distraction arthroplasty for thumb basal joint osteoarthritis: minimum 6.5-year follow-up evaluation. J Hand Surg [Am] 2007;32:23–9.

[19] Burton R, Pellegrini VD. Surgical management of basal joint arthritis of the thumb. Part II. Ligament reconstruction with tendon interposition arthroplasty. J Hand Surg [Am] 1986;11:324–32.

[20] Weilby A. Surgical treatment of osteoarthritis of the carpometacarpal joint of the thumb. Acta Orthop Scand 1971;42:439–40.

[21] Thompson JS. Surgical treatment of trapeziometacarpal arthrosis. Advances in Orthopaedic Surgery 1986;10:105–20.

[22] Kvarnes L, Reikeras O. Osteoarthritis of the carpometacarpal joint of the thumb: an analysis of operative procedures. J Hand Surg [Br] 1985;10:117–20.

[23] Burton RI. Basal joint arthritis: fusion, implant or soft tissue reconstruction? Orthop Clin North Am 1986;17(3):493–502.

[24] Barron OA, Glickel SZ, Eaton RG. Basal joint arthritis of the thumb. J Am Acad Orthop Surg 2000;8:314–23.

[25] Jones NF, Maser BM. Treatment of arthritis of the trapeziometacarpal joint with trapeziectomy and hematoma arthroplasty. Hand Clin 2001;17(2):237–43.

[26] Anwar R, Cohen A, Nicholl JE. The gap after trapeziectomy: a prospective study. J Hand Surg [Br] 2006;31:566–8.

[27] Herren DB, Lehmann O, Simmen BR. Does trapeziectomy destabilize the carpus? J Hand Surg [Br] 1998;23:676–9.

[28] Lins RE, Gelberman RH, McKeown L, et al. Basal joint arthritis: trapeziectomy with ligament reconstruction and tendon interposition arthroplasty. J Hand Surg [Am] 1996;21:202–9.

Treatment of Advanced CMC Joint Disease: Trapeziectomy and Implant Arthroplasty (Silastic–Metal–Synthetic Allograft)

Brandon E. Earp, MD

Department of Orthopaedic Surgery, Brigham and Women's Hospital, 75 Francis Street, Boston, MA 02115, USA

Osteoarthritis of the basal joint of the thumb is a common and frequently debilitating condition, most often affecting middle-aged women. Non-operative treatment with activity modification, splinting, oral anti-inflammatory medication, and intra-articular steroid injection frequently leads to acceptable control of symptoms. If non-operative treatment fails, many surgical techniques have been described for management of symptomatic advanced degenerative joint changes. These include excision of the trapezium alone [1–6], ligament reconstruction with or without inter-position graft [1,7–23], arthrodesis [24–29], and multiple arthroplasty options using with a wide variety of biologic and synthetic implants, including silastic prostheses [6,30–45], metal prostheses [46–53], and allograft interpositions [54,55]. With most of these reconstructive options, satisfactory relief of pain and restoration of function can be achieved. Successful and durable results have been achieved with ligament reconstruction with or without tendon interposition, but concerns about loss of pinch strength due to shortening or instability with trapeziectomy have lead to the de-velopment and design of prosthetic solutions that may aid in maintaining the length of the thumb ray, which may provide greater pinch strength and longevity.

This article will review the literature related to various arthroplasty options for advanced disease. Treatment decisions must clearly be tempered by the surgeon's experience, the patient's goals and expectations, and the extent of degenerative disease.

E-mail address: bearp@partners.org

Silastic

Implant arthroplasty for the treatment of trapeziometacarpal arthritis first began in the 1960's when Swanson and Niebauer each inde-pendently introduced trapeziectomy with silicone implant arthroplasty as a new option for man-agement of symptomatic arthritic disease [39,42]. Their techniques seemed to address and theoreti-cally avoid the issues of stiffness and nonunion found with arthrodesis, and the shortening and in-stability noticed after trapeziectomy. Early results revealed good pain relief, restoration of strength, and maintenance of the thumb length [42,56].

Subsequent dorsoradial subluxation of the implant became a recognized problem and was postulated to be secondary to design as well as technical errors, which lead to changes in both the implant and surgical technique. The importance of adequate bone resection, proper seating of the implant, preservation of the joint capsule, and proper management of the deforming forces due to metacarpophalangeal joint hyperextension and first web space contracture was identified [30,42]. Eaton also designed a cannulated implant to use with abductor pollicis longus graft to attempt to provide added stability but unfortunately sublux-ation continued to be a significant complication at early follow-up [30,56].

Longer-term follow-up studies also began to reveal implant wear and the resultant bone and soft tissue response to silicone particulate matter [57,58]. Osteolysis and erosions in bone adjacent to the implant were noticed typically more than two years postoperatively and appeared to be pro-gressive. Similar findings were found in adjacent extra-articular bones [57]. These findings were often associated with pain and swelling, and at times lead to further surgery for synovectomy, implant removal, and curettage of lytic defects [57,59]. These outcomes lead to a marked decrease in popularity for the use of silicone implants throughout the hand.

Despite the high rates of silicone synovitis noticed with carpal implants in general, the rates of synovitis following trapezium arthroplasty have not been as significant. Pellegrini and Burton [58] performed a review of 32 silicone implant arthroplasties involving four types of implants used to treat trapeziometacarpal arthritis. At approximately four years follow-up, there was close to 50% loss of implant height, with increased wear along the ulnar border. Subluxation averaged 35% of the width of the prosthesis. The Swanson trapezium implants had more subluxation but less wear (Fig. 1). Sixteen percent came to revision surgery and findings included proliferative synovitis with silicone particulate matter [58]. Despite this, all patients with the diagnosis of rheumatoid arthritis and 75% of patients with osteoarthritis were satisfied with their outcome [58].

More recently, Bezwada and colleagues [60] found 84% good to excellent results at 16.4-year follow-up from silicon implant arthroplasty. Subluxation, implant wear, and bony radiolucencies were not found to correlate with subjective outcomes nor clinical importance. Implant fractures, seen in 6%, could be addressed early with good outcomes. No gross silicone synovitis was noted.

Another retrospective comparative review of silicon implant arthroplasty, resection arthroplasty (with or without ligament reconstruction), and arthrodesis was published by Taylor and colleagues [6] in 2005. They evaluated 83 patients (22 with silicon arthroplasty, 25 with trapezial

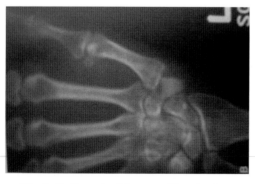

Fig. 1. Radiograph of Swanson silicon implant.

excision with or without ligament reconstruction, and 36 with arthrodesis) at 1–5 year follow-up. Outcome measurements included patient satisfaction, pain, range of motion, tip and key pinch strength, and complications. There were no significant differences between the clinical outcomes of the treatment groups, although they found a higher rate of complications and subsequent re-operation in the fusion group.

Good results can be achieved after silicone trapezium implant arthroplasty, but some studies would suggest that the results may deteriorate with time [61] and at present this technique is recommended for consideration only in low demand patients with rheumatoid arthritis [58]. Other surgical options may achieve equal clinical efficacy in this same population.

Of note, A recent biomechanical study in cadavers performed by Luria and colleagues [62] evaluated the stability of the classic ligament reconstruction with tendon interposition (LRTI) or without tendon interposition compared with a newly developed 1-piece silicone trapezium implant. They found some biomechanical advantages to the implant compared with LRTI, which included decreased axial and radial displacement and maintenance of the trapezial space. These findings were thought to be secondary to the effect of the implant as a spacer. There was significant rotation with the implant perhaps due to implant design, which potentially could be problematic clinically. No clinical data is yet available.

Silicone hemiarthroplasty

Silicone hemiarthroplasty implants were also designed in the 1970's to treat patients with localized trapeziometacarpal arthritis. Kessler [63] created a thin silicone disc that was interposed between the trapezium and metacarpal, but results showed high rates of synovitis and instability. Ashworth and colleagues [64] reported the use of a modified bur-hole cover as a trapeziometacarpal spacer but the outcomes were unsuccessful, and thin silicone implants were subsequently abandoned.

Gore-Tex

The use of Gore-Tex as an interposition spacer has also been attempted. Greenberg and colleagues [65] published their results at an average of 41 months follow-up in 31 patients who underwent 34 expanded polytetrafluoroethylene interpositional (Gore-Tex) arthroplasties. Despite favorable subjective response, radiographic analysis demonstrated a high rate of osteolytic lesions consistent with reactive particulate synovitis. Due to this, the authors recommended that use of this material in this clinical setting be abandoned.

Metallic

As arthroplasty implants and techniques have been refined for larger joints, so too have various attempts been made for developing and improving total joint arthroplasty for trapeziometacarpal arthritis. Many combinations of metallic and polyethylene components have been introduced and continue to be in the experimental stages. Most are ball and socket–type joints with modifications to enhance fixation and motion.

In 1971, de la Caffiniere and Aucouturier [53] introduced a cemented ball and socket type implant to address isolated trapeziometacarpal arthritis due to a variety of etiologies. The implant had a polyethylene cup placed into the trapezium and a stemmed cobalt-chromium ball inserted into the shaft of the thumb metacarpal (Fig. 2). Early findings were reported in 1979, which revealed the best results in patients who had the procedure for pain and instability, with less good outcomes for those who complained of stiffness preoperatively [53].

Other papers have addressed longer-term outcomes after use of the Caffiniere prosthesis [66–69]. Sondergaard and colleagues [68] reported on twenty patients (22 arthroplasties) at a median 9 year follow-up, where 82% of the prostheses were still in place and three had been revised

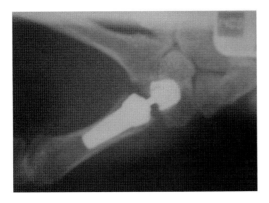

Fig. 2. Radiograph of implanted de la Caffinière prosthesis.

because of aseptic loosening. Good functional results were maintained over this time frame. Nicholas and Calderwood [67] reported a ten-year follow-up of 20 arthroplasties performed for osteoarthritis, and showed that pain relief and range of motion were satisfactory. One patient had asymptomatic radiolucencies noted on radiographic studies. Two patients had experienced failure of their prostheses; one was thought to be secondary to a technical issue of over-reaming of the trapezium, and the other due to traumatic dislocation. Chakrabarti and colleagues [66] reported an 89% survival rate at 16 years for 93 replacements performed in 71 patients. Note was made of a higher prevalence of aseptic loosening of the trapezial component in working-age men, leading the authors to caution using this prosthesis in that population [66]. Van Cappelle and colleagues reported long-term results of 77 Caffiniere prostheses for osteoarthritis at a mean follow-up of 8.5 years (range 2-16 years). At 16 years, the survival rate was 72%, with a total loosening rate of 44%, half of which required revision. Van Cappelle [69] also found a higher revision rate among men, thought to be due to increased functional demands. They recommended use in women over age 60.

Another type of cemented total joint arthroplasty was developed by Cooney and colleagues [48], in which the ball-and-socket components were reversed. The trapezium component was a metallic implant with a pedestal and with a sphere protruding from the bony surface, and the metacarpal component was a polyethylene-stemmed socket.

Short-term results have been similarly positive to the Caffiniere prosthesis, with quick functional return [48,50,70,71]. Cooney and colleagues [48] noted that 36% of the implants in their cohort developed heterotopic bone postoperatively, which negatively affected patient outcome, and they therefore recommended that heterotopic bone noted preoperatively may be a contraindication to this type of arthroplasty. Other contraindications included adjacent joint arthrodesis, which has been shown to lead to rapid loosening of the components [48].

Due to the high loosening rate of cemented trapeziometacarpal arthroplasty, there has been a decline in popularity of these implants [40]. Design changes to the de la Caffiniere prosthesis have been ongoing in attempts to reduce the incidence of metacarpal loosening, but clinical results are not yet available.

Published data in the past few years is more optimistic. Badia and Sambandam [72] reported in 2006 on 25 elderly patients (26 thumbs) who underwent cemented ball-and-socket CMC arthroplasty using the using the Braun-Cutter prosthesis (SBI/Avanta Orthopaedics, San Diego, CA) for stage III and IV trapeziometacarpal disease. At an average of 59 month follow-up, thumb abduction averaged 60° and thumb opposition to the base of the small finger was present. The average pinch strength was 85% of the unaffected side. One patient had posttraumatic loosening, which was revised with satisfactory results. Final follow-up radiographic evaluation did not show signs of implant loosening. 24 of the 25 patients were pain free. They recommended this technique for the treatment of advanced stage thumb CMC osteoarthritis in older patients with low activity demands [72].

Other types of implants have also been developed and marketed for isolated trapeziometacarpal arthritis (stage II and III), including hemiarthroplasties and metallic interposition implants.

Swanson developed a titanium hemiarthroplasty in 1985 with an uncemented stemmed metacarpal implant. In 1997, his group published the outcomes of 105 Swanson titanium condylar implants at an average follow-up of 5 years. At early (6 months) follow-up, they reported increased motion and strength, evidence of bone remodeling, and no significant implant instability. 5-year follow-up also demonstrated no evidence of wear [73].

Athwal and colleagues [74] published their results in 2004 with the use of the Orthosphere (Wright Medical Technology, Arlington, TN), a spherical zirconia implant designed to be inserted after hemispheric reaming of the thumb metacarpal base and trapezium. Seven patients received this implant. At an average 33 month follow-up, six of the seven implants had subsided into the trapezium, with resultant pain and weakness in those patients. This subsidence led to revision surgery involving ligament reconstruction and tendon interposition (LRTI) in five of the seven patients. The authors no longer use the device.

Other currently available options include the Ascension CMC (Ascension Orthopaedics, Inc, Austin, TX), which is a semiconstrained hemiarthroplasty device, recommended for use with an additional stabilization procedure if preoperative instability exists. A similar device is the Pyrohemisphere (Ascension Orthopaedics, Inc, Austin, TX), also a cementless hemiarthroplasty, which does require reaming of the trapezium. Some surgeons have discussed concerns about postoperative instability and dislocation necessitating revision surgery with these implants, thus caution should be exercised and meticulous technique used until long-term data is available.

Synthetic allograft

Artelon

Artelon (Artimplant AB, Sweden) is a T-shaped interpositional spacer made of degradable polyurethaneurea designed to be inserted between the thumb metacarpal base and the trapezium for isolated thumb trapeziometacarpal arthritis. The horizontal portion of the "T" is meant to stabilize the joint.

Nilsson and colleagues [55] reported on 15 patients in a semi-randomized controlled trial. 10 patients who received the Artelon spacer were compared with 5 others who received trapezium resection and abductor pollicis longus stabilization. At three year follow-up, all patients were pain-free and those in the spacer group demonstrated increased key pinch and tripod pinch. They also analyzed a biopsy specimen obtained from one patient at 6 months postoperatively, which showed incorporation of the spacer without signs of foreign body reaction. To date, there is no long-term data available and no studies have documented the success of revision surgery following this procedure.

GRAFTJACKET

Adams and colleagues [54] have described a technique of arthroscopic debridement and interposition arthroplasty of the trapeziometacarpal joint for patient with stage II and II disease. They interposed a commercially available acellular dermal matrix allograft (GRAFTJACKET) between the arthritic metacarpal base and the distal trapezium. In their cohort, all patients had some symptomatic relief and 94% were partially or completely satisfied. 70% of their patients had none or mild difficulty in performing activities of daily living.

Our group (Brandon E. Earp, MD, P. Blazar, B. Simmons, unpublished data, 2007) is currently investigating the use of GRAFTJACKET allograft versus flexor carpi radialis interposition graft with trapezium resection for trapeziometacarpal disease and early results would indicate that the matrix is safe and effective with no significant differences between the groups, but final data are not yet available.

Due to the lack of significant long-term data with these products, appropriate patient education, careful technique, and surgeon discretion is advised when deciding to use them.

Summary

A wide variety of arthroplasty options exist for symptomatic trapeziometacarpal arthritis. Silicone implants have been associated with implant wear, synovitis, and osteolysis. This may not correlate directly with patient satisfaction or clinical relevance but based on clinical data, their use should be limited to low demand patients with rheumatoid arthritis, and other options exist which may provide similar or better results in this same population. Metallic implant arthroplasty has advanced with progressive improvements to address short-comings and failures of prior generation implants. Subsidence, instability, and implant loosening have all been reported with these types of prostheses and have decreased their popularity. Newer changes to the implants may acceptably address these concerns, but caution should be exercised in patient selection and operative technique. Newer synthetic allografts are also on the market to be used as interposition options. No long-term data or larger-scale studies are available to date, and appropriate patient education and surgeon discretion should be undertaken when deciding if and when to use them.

References

[1] Davis TR, Brady O, Barton NJ, et al. Trapeziectomy alone with tendon interposition or with ligament reconstruction? J Hand Surg [Br] 1997;22:689–94.

[2] Davis TR, Brady O, Dias JJ. Excision of the trapezium for osteoarthritis of the trapeziometacarpal joint: a study of the benefit of ligament reconstruction or tendon interposition. J Hand Surg [Am] 2004;29:1069–77.

[3] Gibbons CE, Gosal HS, Choudri AH, et al. Trapeziectomy for basal thumb joint osteoarthritis: 3- to 19-year follow-up. Int Orthop 1999;23:216–8.

[4] Varley GW, Calvey J, Hunter JB, et al. Excision of the trapezium for osteoarthritis at the base of the thumb. J Bone Joint Surg Br 1994;76:964–8.

[5] Amadio PC. A comparison of fusion, trapeziectomy, and silastic replacement for the treatment of osteoarthritis of the trapeziometacarpal joint. J Hand Surg [Br] 2005;30:331–2.

[6] Taylor EJ, Desari K, D'Arcy JC, et al. A comparison of fusion, trapeziectomy and silastic replacement for the treatment of osteoarthritis of the trapeziometacarpal joint. J Hand Surg [Br] 2005;30(1):45–9.

[7] Eaton RG, Littler JW. Ligament reconstuction for the painful thumb carpometacarpal joint. J Bone Joint Surg Am 1973;55:1655–66.

[8] Burton RI. Basal joint arthrosis of the thumb. Orthop Clin North Am 1973;4:347–8.

[9] Burton RI, Pellegrini VD Jr. Surgical management of basal joint arthritis of the thumb: part II. Ligament reconstruction with tendon interposition arthroplasty. J Hand Surg [Am] 1986;11:324–32.

[10] Thompson JS. Surgical treatment of trapeziometacarpal arthrosis. Adv Orthop Surg 1986;10:105–20.

[11] Weilby A. Tendon interposition arthroplasty of the first carpo-metacarpal joint. J Hand Surg [Br] 1988;13:421–5.

[12] Kleinman WB, Eckemode JF. Tendon suspension sling arthroplasty for thumb trapezioaaqetacarpal arthritis. J Hand Surg [Am] 1991;16:983–91.

[13] De Smet L, Sioen W, Spaepen D, et al. Treatment of basal joint arthritis of the thumb: trapeziectomy with or without tendon interposition/ligament reconstruction. Hand Surg 2004;9:5–9.

[14] Barron OA, Eaton RG. Save the trapezium: double interposition arthroplasty for the treatment of stage IV disease of the basal joint. J Hand Surg [Am] 1998; 23:196–204.

[15] Dell PC, Muniz RB. Interposition arthroplasty of the trapeziometacarpal joint for osteoarthritis. Clin Orthop 1987;220:27–34.

[16] Eaton RG, Glickel SZ, Littler JW. Tendon interpositionarthroplasty for degenerative arthritis of the trapeziometacarpal joint of the thumb. J Hand Surg [Am] 1985;10:645–54.

[17] Froimson AI. Tendon interposition arthroplasty of carpometacarpaljoint of the thumb. Hand Clin 1987;3:489–505.

[18] Imaeda T, Cooney WP, Niebur GL, et al. Kinematics of the trapeziometacarpal joint: a biomechanical analysis comparing tendon interposition arthroplasty and total joint arthroplasty. J Hand Surg [Am] 1996;21:544–53.

[19] Kleven T, Russwurm H, Finsen V. Tendon interposition arthroplasty for basal joint arthrosis. 38 thumbs followed for 4 years. Acta Orthop Scand 1996;67:575–7.

[20] Menon J. Partial trapeziectomy and interpositional arthroplasty for trapeziometacarpal osteoarthritis of the thumb. J Hand Surg [Br] 1995;20:700–6.

[21] Menon J, Schoene HR, Hohl JC. Trapeziometacarpal arthritis-results of tendon interpositional arthroplasty. J Hand Surg [Am] 1981;6:442–6.

[22] Mureau MA, Rademaker RP, Verhaar JA, et al. Tendon interposition arthroplasty versus arthrodesis for the treatment of trapeziometacarpal

arthritis: a retrospective comparative follow-up study. J Hand Surg [Am] 2001;26:869–76.

[23] Nylen S, Juhlin LJ, Lugnegard H. Weilby tendon interposition arthroplasty for osteoarthritis of the trapezial joints. J Hand Surg [Br] 1987;12:68–72.

[24] Amadio PC, De Silva SP. Comparison of the results of trapeziometacarpal arthrodesis and arthroplasty in men with osteoarthritis of the trapeziometacarpal joint. Ann Chir Main Memb Super 1990;9:358–63.

[25] Bamberger HB, Stern PJ, Kiefhaber TR, et al. Trapeziometacarpal joint arthrodesis: a functional evaluation. J Hand Surg [Am] 1992;17:605–11.

[26] Carroll RE. Arthrodesis of the carpometacarpal joint of the thumb. A review of patients with a long postoperative period. Clin Orthop 1987;220: 106–10.

[27] Damen A, Dijsktra T, van der Lei B, et al. Long-term results of arthrodesis of the carpometacarpal joint of the thumb. Scand J Plast Reconstr Surg Hand Surg 2001;35:407–13.

[28] Hartigan BJ, Stern PJ, Kiefhaber TR. Thumb carpometacarpal osteoarthritis: arthrodesis compared with ligament recon reconstruction and tendon interposition. J Bone Joint Surg Am 2001; 83:1470–8.

[29] Lisanti M, Rosati M, Spagnolli G, et al. Trapeziometacarpal joint arthrodesis for osteoarthritis. Results of power staple fixation. J Hand Surg [Br] 1997;22:576–9.

[30] Swanson AB, deGroot Swanson G, Watermeier JJ. Trapezium implant arthroplasty. Long-term evaluation of 150 cases. J Hand Surg 1981;6:125–41.

[31] Amadio PC, Millender LH, Smith RJ. Silicone spacer or tendon spacer for trapezium resection arthroplasty—comparison of results. J Hand Surg 1982;7:237–44.

[32] Braun RM. Stabilization of Silastic implant arthroplasty at the trapeziometacarpal joint. Clin Orthop 1976;121:263–70.

[33] Eiken O, Necking LE. Silicone rubber implants for arthrosis of the scaphotrapezial trapezoidal joint. Scand J Plast Reconstr Surg 1983;17:253–5.

[34] Freeman GR, Honner R. Silastic long term replacement of the trapezium. J Hand Surg [Br] 1992;17: 458–62.

[35] Hay EL, Bomberg BC, Burke C, et al. Results of silicone trapezial implant arthroplasty. J Arthroplasty 1988;3:215–23.

[36] Hofammann DY, Ferlic DC, Clayton ML. Arthroplasty of the basal joint of the thumb using a silicone prosthesis—long-term follow-up. J Bone Joint Surg Am 1987;69:993–7.

[37] Lehmann O, Herren DB, Simmen BR. Comparison of tendon suspension-interposition and silicon spacers in the treatment of degenerative osteoarthritis of the base of the thumb. Ann Chir Main Memb Super 1998;17:25–30.

[38] Lovell ME, Nuttall D, Trail IA, et al. A patient-reported comparison of trapeziectomy with Swanson Silastic implant or sling ligament reconstruction. J Hand Surg [Br] 1999;24:453–5.

[39] Niebauer JJ, Shaw JL, Doren WW. Silicone-Dacron hinge prosthesis. Design, evaluation, and application. Ann Rheum Dis 1969;28(Suppl):56–8.

[40] Ruffin RA, Rayan GM. Treatment of trapeziometacarpal arthritis with silastic and metallic implant arthroplasty. Hand Clin 2001;17:245–53.

[41] Swanson AB. Finger joint replacement by silicone rubber implants and the concept of implant fixation by encapsulation. Ann Rheum Dis 1969;28(Suppl): 47–55.

[42] Swanson AB. Disabling arthritis at the base of the thumb: treatment by resection of the trapezium and flexible (silicone) implant arthroplasty. J Bone Joint Surg Am 1972;54:456–71.

[43] Tagil M, Kopylov P. Swanson versus APL arthroplasty in the treatment of osteoarthritis of the trapeziometacarpal joint: a prospective and randomized study in 26 patients. J Hand Surg [Br] 2002;27:452–6.

[44] Weilby A, Sondorf J. Results following removal of silicone trapezium metacarpal implants. J Hand Surg 1978;3:154–6.

[45] Wood VE. Unusual complication of a silicone implant arthroplasty at the base of the thumb. J Hand Surg [Br] 1984;9:67–8.

[46] Cooney WE. Arthroplasty of the thumb axis. In: Morrey BF, Cooney WP, Chao EYS, editors. Joint replacement arthroplasty. New York: Churchill Livingstone; 1991. p. 173–94.

[47] de la Caffiniere JY. L'art/culation traozoradtacarpiennc approche bio-mdcmfique et appareil ligamentaire. Arch Anat Pathol (Paris) 1970;18: 277–84.

[48] Cooney WP, Linscheid Rio, Askew LJ. Total arthroplasty of the thumb trapeziometacarpal joint. Clin Orthop 1987;220:35–45.

[49] Cooney WP III, Lucca MJ, Chao EY, et al. The kinesiology of the thumb trapeziometacmpal joint. J Bone Joint Surg 1981;63:1371–81.

[50] Braun RM. Total joint replacement at the base of the thumb: preliminary report. J Hand Surg 1982;7: 245–51.

[51] Ledoux P. Cementless totral trapezio-raetacarpal prosthesis. Principle of anchorage. In: Schuind RAn gag, Cooney WP, Garcia-Elias M, editors. Advances in the biomechanics of the hand and wrist. NewYork: Plenum Press; 1994. p. 25–30.

[52] Alnot JY, Saim Laurent Y. Total trapeziometacarpal arthroplasty: report on seventeen cases of degenerative arthritis of the trapeziometacarpal joint. Ann Chir Main 1985;4:11–21.

[53] de la Caffiniere JY, Aucouturier P. Trapeziometacarpal arthroplasty by total prosthesis. Hand 1979; 11:41–6.

[54] Adams JE, Merten SM, Steinmann SP. Arthroscopic interposition arthroplasty of the first carpometacarpal joint. J Hand Surg Eur Vol 2007;32(3):268–74.

[55] Nilsson A, Liljensten E, Bergstrom C, et al. Results from a degradable TMC joint spacer (Artelon) compared with tendon arthroplasty. J Hand Surg [Am] 2005;30:380–9.

[56] Haffajee D. Endoprosthetic replacement of the trapezium for arthrosis in the carpometacarpal joint of the thumb. J Hand Surg [Am] 1977;2: 141–8.

[57] Peimer CA. Long-term complications of trapeziometacarpal silicone arthroplasty. Clin Orthop 1987;220:86–98.

[58] Pellegrini VD Jr, Burton RI. Surgical management of basal joint arthritis of the thumb: I. Long-term results of silicone implant arthroplasty. J Hand Surg [Am] 1986;11:309–24.

[59] Peimer CA, Medige J, Eckert BS, et al. Reactive synovitis after silicone arthroplasty. J Hand Surg [Am] 1986;11:624–38.

[60] Bezwada HP, Sauer ST, Hankins ST, et al. Long-term results of trapeziometacarpal silicone arthroplasty. J Hand Surg [Am] 2002;27:409–17.

[61] Sollerman C, Herrlin K, Abrahamson SO, et al. Silastic replacement of the trapezium for arthrosis: a 12-year follow-up study. J Hand Surg [Br] 1988; 13:426–9.

[62] Luria S, Waitayawinyu T, Nemechek N, et al. Biomechanic analysis of trapeziectomy, ligament reconstruction with tendon interposition, and tie-in trapezium implant arthroplasty for thumb carpometacarpal arthritis: a cadaver study. J Hand Surg [Am] 2007;32(5):697–706.

[63] Kessler F, Epstein M, Culver J, et al. Proplast stabilized stemless trapezium implant. J Hand Surg [Am] 1984;9:227–31.

[64] Ashworth CR, Blatt G, Chuinard RG, et al. Silicone-rubber interposition arthroplasty of the carpometacarpal joint of the thumb. J Hand Surg [Am] 1977;2:345–57.

[65] Greenberg JA, Mosher JF, Fatti JF. X-ray changes after expanded polytetrafluoroethylene (Gore-Tex) interpositional arthroplasty. J Hand Surg [Am] 1997;22:658–63.

[66] Chakrabarti AJ, Robinson AH, Gallagher P. De la Caffiniere thumb carpometacarpal replacements: 93 cases at 6 to 16 years follow-up. J Hand Surg [Br] 1997;22:695–8.

[67] Nicholas RM, Calderwood JW. De la Caffiniere arthroplasty for basal thumb joint osteoarthritis. J Bone Joint Surg Br 1992;74:309–12.

[68] Sondergaard L, Konradsen L, Rechnagel K. Long-term follow-up of the cemented Caffiniere prosthesis for trapeziometacarpal arthroplasty. J Hand Surg [Br] 1991;16:428–30.

[69] van Cappelle HG, Elzenga P, van Horn JR. Long-term results and loosening analysis of de la Caffiniere replacements of the trapeziometacarpal joint. J Hand Surg 1999;24:476–82.

[70] Ferrari B, Steffee AD. Trapeziometacarpal total joint replacement using the Steffee prosthesis. J Bone Joint Surg Am 1986;68:1177–84.

[71] McGovern RM, Shin AY, Beckenbaugh RD, et al. Long-term results of cemented Steffe arthroplasty of the thumb metacarpophalangeal joint. J Hand Surg [Am] 2001;26:115–22.

[72] Badia A, Sambandam SN. Total joint arthroplasty in the treatment of advanced stages of thumb carpometacarpal joint osteoarthritis. J Hand Surg [Am] 2006;31:1605–14.

[73] Swanson AB, de Groot Swanson G, DeHeer DH, et al. Carpal bone titanium implant arthroplasty: 10 years' experience. Clin Orthop Relat Res 1997; 342:46–58.

[74] Athwal GS, Chenkin J, King GJ, et al. Early failures with a spheric interposition arthroplasty of the thumb basal joint. J Hand Surg [Am] 2004;29: 1080–4.

HAND
CLINICS

Hand Clin 24 (2008) 285–294

Treatment of Advanced Carpometacarpal Joint Disease: Arthrodesis

Julia A. Kenniston, MD[a],*, David J. Bozentka, MD[b]

[a]Department of Orthopaedic Surgery, Hospital of the University of Pennsylvania, Silverstein 2, 3400 Spruce Street, Philadelphia, PA 19104, USA
[b]Department of Orthopaedic Surgery, University of Pennsylvania, Penn Presbyterian Medical Center, 39th and Market Street, Philadelphia, PA 19104, USA

The thumb carpometacarpal (CMC) joint, also known as the trapeziometacarpal (TM) joint, is a common location affected by osteoarthritis. This disease process causes disabling pain at the base of the thumb and progresses to deformity and limitations in motion. The affected hand may additionally become weak and clumsy, thereby affecting the quality of life for patients. Due to the importance of this joint in activities of daily living, it has become the site in the upper extremity that most frequently requires surgical intervention for osteoarthritis.

Treatment for degenerative osteoarthritis of the thumb CMC joint begins with nonoperative management. However, if patients continue to have symptoms despite conservative treatment, a variety of surgical options are available. The surgical technique used is largely dependent on radiographic and clinical criteria. One of these techniques is arthrodesis, a valuable tool in treating isolated thumb CMC arthritis and producing pain relief, stability, and maintenance of strength and functional motion of the thumb.

Etiology

Symptomatic thumb CMC degenerative arthritis can be idiopathic, posttraumatic, or associated with congenital ligamentous laxity [1–4]. Historically, this disease has predominantly affected postmenopausal women without a clear etiology

defined. Radiographically, it has been shown that 25% of postmenopausal women have evidence of degenerative changes in the TM joint, although only one in three have symptoms [5].

Posttraumatic arthritis may also cause thumb CMC pain and is generally seen in males after suffering a prior Bennett or Rolando fracture. In addition, younger women with generalized ligamentous laxity and joint hypermobility may also be affected by TM arthritis.

Anatomy and biomechanics

The articulation of the thumb metacarpal and trapezium form a biconcave saddle-shaped joint that can function in many different planes. The ability of the thumb to flex, extend, abduct, adduct, and oppose depends on muscular activity and lack of bony constraints. Due to the limited osseous congruence, which could potentially limit motion, the TM joint relies on static ligamentous restraints to maintain alignment. The volar oblique ligament, also referred to as the "beak ligament," is considered the primary stabilizer of the TM joint and functions as the primary restraint against dorsal translation of the metacarpal on the trapezium [6]. It is postulated that pathologic ligamentous laxity of the beak ligament increases the risk of degenerative changes seen in the CMC joint of the thumb due to destabilization of the joint.

Biomechanics and pathoanatomy

The thumb joint requires dexterity, stability, and strength to withstand the forces applied during

* Corresponding author.
 E-mail address: julia.kenniston@uphs.upenn.edu (J.A. Kenniston).

0749-0712/08/$ - see front matter. Published by Elsevier Inc.
doi:10.1016/j.hcl.2008.03.006

hand.theclinics.com

pinch or grip. The joint compression force at the TM interface is 12 times the applied force at the tips of the thumb and index finger during simple pinch. In addition, the extrinsic and intrinsic tendons of the thumb can sustain forces of up to 30 times that of the applied force with the same simple pinch maneuver [7].

The thumb is able to perform palmar abduction, palmar adduction, extension, and flexion, as well as rotation about the long axis of the thumb metacarpal [4]. The functional position of the hand (flexion/adduction) causes compression forces localized to the volar articular surfaces while opposition of the thumb with axial rotation results in increased shear forces at the joint surface [8].

Clinical presentation

Most patients suffering from TM arthritis present with insidious onset of pain at the basal joint of the thumb or thenar eminence, weakness, and activity-related pain, particularly with pinch or grip maneuvers. As the disease advances, patients may complain of pain at rest and have instability or deformity. On physical examination, it is important to compare the involved side with the contralateral unaffected hand. There may be dorsoradial prominence of the basal joint from subluxation, joint inflammation, or osteophytes. In the later stages of the disease, there may be an adduction deformity from shortening of the adductor pollicis with compensatory hyperextension of the metacarpophalangeal (MP) joint.

Radiographs

Plain radiographs should be obtained to better characterize the extent of the degenerative changes. CT and MRI are rarely required for the diagnosis of thumb CMC arthritis. Only 33% of radiographic TM arthritis is symptomatic [5]. Therefore, treatment should not be based solely on radiographic evidence. Radiographs are useful to confirm the diagnosis of arthritis and to localize joint involvement. With thumb CMC arthritis, radiographic staging is a valuable tool in determining the most appropriate treatment method.

The views obtained for assessment of CMC arthritis of the thumb include posteroanterior, lateral, oblique, and dynamic stress views. The Roberts view is an anterior-posterior radiograph with the hand in hyperpronation. This view allows

visualization of all four trapezial articulations. Stress views involve posteroanterior projections of bilateral basal joints with simultaneous pressure exerted by the adjacent radial borders of the thumb tips [9]. The stress view radiographs are most useful when the nonstress views appear normal. The force exerted on the CMC joint may reveal TM hypermobility or instability that is not evident in other views [10].

The four stages of thumb CMC arthritis were first described by Eaton and Littler in 1973 [9]. Stage I is characterized by either a normal joint appearance or a slightly widened TM joint. The widening of the joint may be secondary to inflammatory synovitis with effusion or ligamentous laxity. Stress views are most helpful in this stage to evaluate for TM joint subluxation. Stage II reveals narrowing of the joint space with osteophyte formation or joint debris that is less than 2 mm in diameter. Stage III has progression of degenerative changes with sclerosis, subchondral cyst formation, and osteophytes or loose bodies that are greater than 2 mm in diameter. The scaphotrapezial (ST) joint is preserved in stage III. With stage IV disease, there is evidence of severe degenerative changes in the TM joint along with involvement of the ST joint (Fig. 1).

Treatment options

Management of CMC arthritis should always begin with nonoperative treatment regimens before attempting surgical intervention. Initial treatment consists of anti-inflammatory medication and activity modification, such as resting the affected extremity, using larger instruments, modifying the need for forceful pinch activities, or increasing the use of the contralateral hand. Immobilization of the extremity for a limited amount of time may also reduce symptoms. In a study evaluating the use of thumb spica splints for CMC arthritis, 55% of patients reported improvement in symptom severity after continuous use of a long thumb spica for 3 to 4 weeks [11]. Corticosteroid injections can also be used as an adjuvant in the management of early-stage CMC arthritis. For stage I arthritis, a single steroid injection and 3 weeks of splinting has been associated with long-term pain relief [12].

The majority of patients achieve pain relief from thumb CMC arthritis with conservative management, such as activity modification, anti-inflammatories, short-term immobilization, and steroid injections [13]. For patients who have

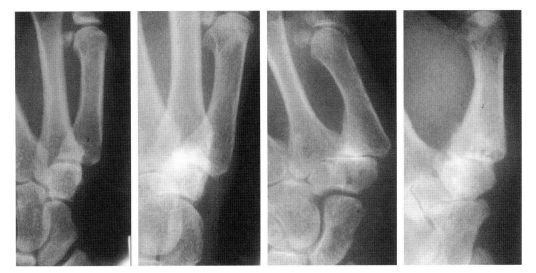

Fig. 1. Staging for CMC arthritis. Stage I (*far left*) with normal appearance. This stage may have joint space widening from synovitis or laxity of ligaments. Stage II (*second from left*) shows narrowing of the joint space with osteophytes or loose bodies less than 2 mm in diameter. Stage III (*second from right*) reveals sclerosis of the articular surfaces with subchondral cyst formation and osteophytes or loose bodies greater than 2 mm in diameter and a normal ST joint. Stage IV (*far right*) displays pantrapezial arthritis. (*From* Barron OA, Eaton RG. Save the trapezium: double interposition arthroplasty for the treatment of stage IV disease of the basal joint. J Hand Surg [Am] 1998;2:197; with permission.)

persistent symptoms despite nonoperative management, surgical intervention should be considered.

Operative management based on radiographic staging

The goal of surgery for thumb CMC arthritis is to minimize pain while maintaining thumb strength, motion, and function. Multiple surgical treatment options are available if patients fail nonoperative treatment. Radiographic staging of CMC arthritis assists in determining the proper surgical technique necessary for optimal results.

The treatment for stage I disease has typically been directed toward correcting the TM joint laxity or to redistribute the TM contact and load. The two methods commonly used at this stage are volar ligament reconstruction or metacarpal osteotomy. Ligament reconstruction and capsular reinforcement may be performed using the flexor carpi radialis, abductor pollicis longus, extensor carpi radialis longus, or extensor carpi radialis brevis. Eaton and colleagues [14] described the use of flexor carpi radialis for reconstruction of the volar ligament with resultant stabilization of the TM joint and found good to

excellent results in 95% of patients with stage I or II disease at a 7-year follow-up. Metacarpal osteotomies are used to alter the force distribution at the TM joint and have been found to be successful in early stage arthritis [15,16].

Stage II and stage III arthritis can be treated in a variety of ways. However, it is essential to ensure that the arthritis is localized to the TM joint and does not include adjacent joints. The treatment method chosen is based on the severity of symptoms as well as the functional demands of the patient. Potential surgical options for stage II and III disease include trapeziectomy with or without ligament reconstruction and tendon interposition (LRTI), interpositional arthroplasty, TM joint replacement, or TM fusion.

Finally, the surgical management for stage IV (pantrapezial) arthritis includes trapeziectomy with or without LRTI, interpositional arthroplasty, and joint arthroplasty. Arthrodesis is not recommended for pantrapezial arthritis or adjacent joint arthritis because functional motion of the thumb depends on increased motion at adjacent joints to compensate for the lack of motion at the fused TM joint. Additionally, for pantrapezial arthritis, the TM fusion addresses only one of the involved joints and may adversely affect the other articulation sites.

Trapeziometacarpal joint arthrodesis

Patient selection

Arthrodesis of the CMC joint of the thumb has proven to be a useful tool for the treatment of stage II and stage III disease. It has been shown to provide pain relief and result in a strong, stable, and functional hand at the expense of full mobility of the CMC joint. Patient selection is important in the decision-making process for a successful outcome. Previously, this surgery was recommended in young high-demand patients and was not recommended for patients over 50 because older patients were presumed to be prone to progression of pantrapezial arthritis postoperatively [17]. More recently, arthrodesis has been successfully used in treating the older patient [18].

The most important selection criterion for arthrodesis is localized TM arthritic changes without degenerative changes in the ST or MP joint. The patient needs full MP and interphalangeal range of motion as the limited CMC joint after fusion is compensated by the MP, interphalangeal, and ST joints.

Arthrodesis is also an alternative to arthroplasty for patients with soft tissue laxity that will not allow stability of the joint after replacement. In these patients, there is a high probability of dislocation or mechanical failure of the arthroplasty. Therefore fusion may be a better option to reduce the risk of complications postoperatively.

Arthrodesis is not recommended in patients with arthritis in adjacent joints or in patients whose lifestyle requires a mobile thumb joint. As mentioned previously, adjacent joint arthritis may further limit thumb motion postfusion, resulting in unacceptable functional motion. Also, occupational and recreational activities must be taken into consideration because fusion decreases the mobility of the thumb joint despite the compensatory motion at adjacent joints and may interfere with certain activities that require a fully mobile thumb.

Technique

There are multiple surgical techniques for arthrodesis of the CMC joint [19,20]. However, the position of fusion is standard. The thumb is placed in the "position of a clenched fist" in which the distal phalanx of the thumb comfortably rests on the middle phalanx of the index finger with a fully clenched fist [1,21]. Specifically, this position is 30° to 40° of palmar abduction, 35° of radial abduction, 15° of pronation, and 10° of extension [22].

Surgical positioning of the patient is supine with the use of a hand table. A tourniquet is used above the elbow to limit bleeding into the surgical field. General or regional anesthesia is performed. After exsanguinations of the limb, the tourniquet is elevated to 100 mm Hg above the systolic pressure. A longitudinal incision over the first dorsal compartment is made between the extensor pollicis brevis and abductor pollicis longus tendon from the midshaft of the thumb metacarpal to the proximal radial styloid process. Alternatively, the incision can be made between the extensor pollicis brevis and the extensor pollicis longus. In either approach, branches from the dorsal sensory radial nerve and the radial artery should be identified and protected.

The TM joint is sharply exposed longitudinally via a capsulotomy reflecting the periosteum, capsule, and portions of the abductor pollicis longus insertion from its attachments (Fig. 2). This flap should be in continuity to allow for repair at the end of the fusion. The peritrapezial joints are not routinely exposed. However, if there is concern regarding the status of the ST joint, the incision can be extended proximally using care to protect the dorsal branch of the radial artery. The ST joint should be directly visualized at this time to determine the best technique to use. If there is any evidence of ST arthritis, the arthrodesis should be abandoned and an alternate technique should be performed.

The base of the thumb metacarpal is then delivered into the incision by flexing and adduction the shaft. The articular cartilage and

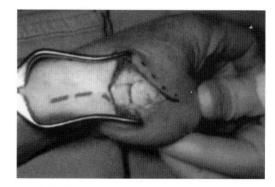

Fig. 2. Exposure of TM joint. (*From* Hanel DP, Condit DP. Thumb carpometacarpal joint fusion with plate and screw fixation. Atlas of the Hand Clinics 1998;3:41–59; with permission.)

eburnated bone are removed from the base of the metacarpal, exposing the underlying cancellous bone. The trapezial surface is prepared in a similar fashion. The articulating surfaces should be molded with the aid of rongeurs, osteotomes, or curettes to create maximum bony contact when the two opposing surfaces are brought together. This often involves maintaining the contour of the TM joint but, in more severe deformities, requires fashioning the bones with a cup-and-cone technique. The thumb is then placed into the position of fusion with the TM joint reapproximated. The surfaces should be reinspected to confirm satisfactory osseous congruence.

There are multiple fixation methods to allow for CMC fusion. The use of Kirschner wires (K-wires) is a common fixation method due to their ease of use. K-wires with a diameter of 0.045 inches are initially placed in the metacarpal while their position is confirmed just exiting the base. The TM joint is then positioned appropriately and compressed manually while the K-wires are driven across the joint to achieve fixation. If three K-wires are used, one wire is parallel to the long axis while the other two wires are crossed at an angle of 15° from the longitudinal plane (Fig. 3). These wires should not extend proximal to the trapezium into the scaphoid except in the case of osteopenic bone when the trapezium does not allow adequate stable fixation. The K-wires are cut below the skin.

If performing arthrodesis with the use of plate and screw fixation, a 0.045- or 0.062-in diameter K-wire may be used for provisional fixation

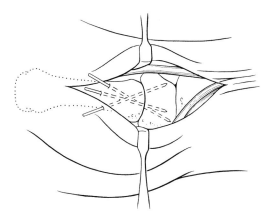

Fig. 3. Arthrodesis with three K-wires. (*From* Schwendeman LJ, Stern PJ. Trapeziometacarpal joint fusion. Atlas of the Hand Clinics 1997;2:169–82; with permission.)

before applying the plate. Various minifragment plates can be used including 2.0-mm or 2.7-mm T plates or minicondylar plates. Minifragment locking plate fixation provides a fixed-angle device that creates a construct that is less prone to toggling and loosening. The hardware is contoured and should be placed on the dorsal surface of the metacarpal slightly offset ulnarly to prevent screws from traversing the trapezio-trapezoid joint. Holes are drilled, measured, and filled with screws of the appropriate size. Intraoperative fluoroscopy is used to monitor screw length and placement (Fig. 4).

Other methods described in the literature have used bone block, tension bands, cerclage wires, staples, or Herbert screws rather than the K-wires or plate and screws for fixation (Fig. 5). These fixation methods may also be combined with bone grafting techniques to enhance fusion.

Bone graft is placed in the areas of poor bony contact. The bone graft is harvested from the distal radius through the floor of the first dorsal compartment. First the extensor retinaculum is incised over the first dorsal compartment and the abductor pollicis longus and extensor pollicis brevis are retracted to expose the distal radius. A cortical window is created in the distal radius and cancellous bone graft is harvested using curettes and packed into the fusion site. Alternatively, a Craig needle biopsy set may be used to harvest the cancellous bone.

The capsule is then repaired over the TM joint and hardware. The tourniquet is deflated and hemostasis is achieved with use of bipolar electrocautery. Nylon sutures are used in a horizontal mattress style to approximate the skin edges and a sterile dressing is applied.

Postoperatively, patients are immobilized in a short-arm thumb-spica and evaluated 5 to 10 days after surgery. An orthoplast thumb-spica splint with the interphalangeal joint free is fabricated for patients with stable fixation and may be removed for bathing. Radiographs are obtained periodically to assess for evidence of fusion. A CT scan is occasionally required to determine consolidation of the joint when radiographs are equivocal. Splint protection is continued until adequate fusion is confirmed clinically and radiographically (Fig. 6). Range-of-motion and strengthening exercises are then instituted. K-wires are removed on average at 6 to 8 weeks postoperatively. The plate fixation is not routinely removed but may become symptomatic related to prominence of the hardware.

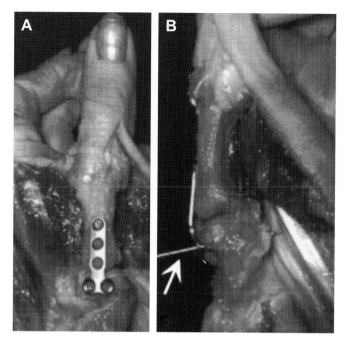

Fig. 4. Plate and screw fixation of TM joint. (*A*) Position for plate fixation of the thumb TM joint. (*B*) Lateral view of plate position for TM fusion. White arrow indicates provisional K-wire fixation. (*From* Hanel DP, Condit DP. Thumb carpometacarpal joint fusion with plate and screw fixation. Atlas of the Hand Clinics 1998;3:41–59; with permission.)

Results

Over the past 40 years, there have been excellent results reported from fusion of the TM joint. Leach and Bolton [1] in 1968 found that 89% of his patients had excellent results with no pain after fusion and immobilization for 10 to 12 weeks. All these patients resumed their normal activities and felt that their operative hand became stronger after surgery. Although there was reduced motion, it did not hinder their function.

Eaton and Littler [21] in 1969 also reported improved hand function in all patients and 92% with pain relief after fusion. Investigators found, however, a 17% nonunion rate, which was asymptomatic. Follow-up analysis up to 11 years postoperatively did not reveal any degenerative changes in adjacent joints.

Grip strength was measured by Stark and colleagues [23] in 1977 and determined to be within 10% of the unaffected contralateral side. This study revealed a 6% nonunion rate and a 3% rate of progression of ST arthritis. The investigators attributed the ST arthritis to an improperly placed K-wire during the time of fusion. Subjectively, all patients had pain relief and felt that the gain in stability and strength compensated for the slight loss in motion.

In a 10-year follow-up study, Cavallazzi and Spreafico [24] found that 56% of the patients had normal pinch power postoperatively and 77% of patients were able to abduct the CMC joint greater than 45° and oppose the thumb to the ring finger. Ninety-eight percent of patients were satisfied after the procedure and 70% were completely pain-free.

Carroll [17] performed fusions on patients under the age of 50 and excluded older patients because he believed the older patients would develop pantrapezial arthritis postoperatively. The arc of palmar abduction and adduction was 20° after surgery. However, despite this limitation, patients had a functional hand due to the increased mobility of the MP and ST joint. No patients had progression of ST degenerative changes.

Alberts and Engkvist [25] had less success with arthrodesis of the first CMC joint as they had only a 60% patient satisfaction rate. The fixation method employed used K-wires or cerclage with bone grafting in 33% of the cases. Twenty-one percent of patients progressed to peritrapezial arthritis and there was a 12% nonunion rate.

Clough and colleagues [26] used a Herbert screw for arthrodesis and immobilized patients for 8 weeks. Although there was a 100% patient

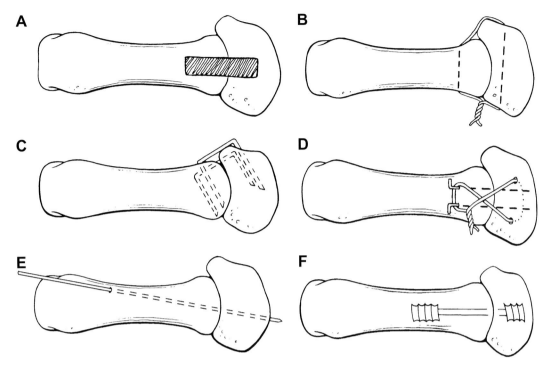

Fig. 5. Methods of carpometacarpal arthrodesis. (*A*) Slotted bone graft. (*B*) Cerclage wiring. (*C*) Staple fixation. (*D*) Tension band wiring. (*E*) K-wire fixation. (*F*) Screw fixation. (*From* Schwendeman LJ, Stern PJ. Trapeziometacarpal joint fusion. Atlas of the Hand Clinics 1997;2:169–82; with permission.)

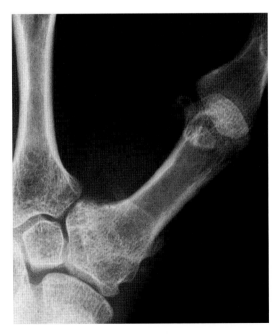

Fig. 6. Fused TM joint. (*From* Fulton DB, Stern PJ. Trapeziometacarpal arthrodesis in primary osteoarthritis: a minimum two-year follow-up study. J Hand Surg [Am] 2001;26:109–14; with permission.)

satisfaction rate and 100% of the patients reported decreased pain compared with preoperatively, there was a 50% nonunion rate determined radiographically.

Functional evaluation after fusion, performed by Bamberger and colleagues [2] in 1992, revealed a 72% decrease in the adduction/adduction arc of motion and a 61% decrease in the flexion/extension arc. Despite this loss of motion, there were minimal subjective functional complaints. In this study, there was an 8% nonunion rate with 5% of patients having ST degenerative changes at an average 4-year follow-up.

Chamay and Piaget-Morerod [3] evaluated 32 TM joint fusions in patients between the ages of 40 and 70 after fixation using tension banding, screws, plates, or staples. Bone grafting was not performed and patients were immobilized for up to 5 weeks. The reoperation rate was 44% for hardware removal due to pain or discomfort and they reported a 12.5% nonunion rate. Forty-four percent of patients complained of the inability to flatten their hand and 41% reported difficulty handling small objects. There was a 4% decrease in grip strength and a 6% decrease in key pinch. Although 90.7% of patients had successful pain relief, only 78.1% were completely satisfied with the results.

Contrary to Carroll's [17] recommendations not to perform CMC fusion in older patients, Fulton supports arthrodesis for symptomatic TM arthritis in older patients. His recommendations are based on his analysis of 49 patients between the ages of 41 and 73 who underwent arthrodesis using K-wires and bone graft for primary osteoarthritis. At an average 7-year follow-up, pain scores were reported as 1.5 on a 10-point scale despite a 12% rate of peritrapezial arthritis and a 7% nonunion rate [18].

Comparison between arthrodesis and other surgical options for carpometacarpal arthritis

Comparisons in treatment options for CMC arthritis support arthrodesis as an excellent option for patients who need a strong, stable CMC joint and are not concerned with the lack of motion. Kvarnes and Reikeras [27] compared fusion to trapeziectomy and arthroplasty and found better strength and stability with fusion. They concluded that fusion is the best surgical option to preserve strength in treating thumb CMC arthritis.

In a review of treatment options, Wolock and colleagues [4] recommended arthrodesis for young heavy-laborers with no ST arthritis who would be able to tolerate the long period of immobilization. He also preferred arthrodesis over arthroplasty in patients with metacarpal subluxation or ligamentous laxity due to the higher risk for dislocation with arthroplasty.

Hartigan and colleagues [28] performed a comparison between LRTI and arthrodesis and found increased lateral pinch strength with fusion. They noted improved thumb motion and the ability to lay the hand flat with LRTI. In general, fusion was used and recommended for young laborers and LRTI for low-demand elderly patients. There was a greater than 90% satisfaction rate with both procedures.

Complications

Overall, the studies assessing arthrodesis for thumb CMC arthritis have reported excellent patient satisfaction with pain relief and a strong, functional hand despite the limitations in CMC range of motion. However the complication rate has been reported as high as 73%. Common complications include nonunion and progression of peritrapezial arthritis. The average reported nonunion rate is 13% [2]. Symptomatic nonunion may be treated with revision arthrodesis or trapezial excision and soft tissue interposition. Progression of peritrapezial arthritis ranges from 0% to 40% [3,24,27]. Other complications include radial sensory neuritis and symptomatic hardware requiring removal.

In their series of 26 arthrodeses, Froseth and Stern [29] reported a higher complication rate and more frequent surgery following plate and screw fixation compared with pin fixation. They noted one of the most common complications was hardware malposition, including screw penetration into the trapezial-trapezoid joint. However, this complication did not affect patient satisfaction or pain.

The main disadvantages of thumb CMC arthrodesis include the long postoperative immobilization period, the inability to lay the hand flat, and loss of motion. Although there is a decreased arc of motion from the TM joint, the motion is compensated by the MP and ST joints. There is increased motion by 75% at the MP joint and 25% at the ST joint to allow patients to have a functional thumb range of motion postfusion [30]. Despite the potential complications and disadvantages of the surgery, the patient satisfaction rate after fusion is generally greater than 90%.

Summary

Advanced thumb CMC arthritis is a disease that largely affects postmenopausal women but may also affect younger patients after intra-articular fractures of the CMC joint or ligamentous laxity. The treatment for this disease begins with nonoperative management consisting of activity modification, nonsteroidal anti-inflammatories, temporary immobilization, and steroid injections. If patients fail conservative management, multiple surgical options are available. The recommended procedure is largely based on clinical symptoms, radiographic staging of the disease, and surgeon and patient preference. Arthrodesis of the TM joint may be used for stage II or stage III disease in the high-demand patient. This surgery creates a pain-free, strong, stable thumb at the expense of full range of motion. Despite the potential complications and disadvantages of the surgery (eg, nonunion and the inability to lay the hand flat), there is a high patient satisfaction rate. Arthrodesis remains an excellent option for patients with isolated CMC arthritis who need a pain-free and strong thumb.

References

[1] Leach RE, Bolton PE. Arthritis of the carpometacarpal joint of the thumb: results of arthrodesis. J Bone Joint Surg Am 1968;50:1171–7.

[2] Bamberger HG, Stern PJ, Kiefhaber TR, et al. Trapeziometacarpal joint arthrodesis: a functional evaluation. J Hand Surg [Am] 1992;17:605–11.

[3] Chamay A, Piaget-Morerod F. Arthrodesis of the trapeziometacarpal joint. J Hand Surg [Br] 1994; 19:489–97.

[4] Wolock BS, Moore JR, Weiland AJ. Arthritis of the basal joint of the thumb: a critical analysis of treatment options. J Arthroplasty 1989;4:65–78.

[5] Armstrong AL, Hunter JB, Davis TR. The prevalence of degenerative arthritis of the base of the thumb in post-menopausal women. J Hand Surg [Br] 1994;19:340–1.

[6] Pellegrini VD Jr. Osteoarthritis of the trapeziometacarpal joint: the pathophysiology of articular cartilage degeneration. I. Anatomy and pathology of the aging joint. J Hand Surg [Am] 1991;16:967–74.

[7] Cooney WP III, Chao EY. Biomechanical analysis of static forces in the thumb during hand function. J Bone Joint Surg Am 1977;59:27–36.

[8] Pellegrini VD Jr, Olcott CW, Hollenberg G. Contact patterns in the trapeziometacarpal joint: the role of the palmar beak ligament. J Hand Surg [Am] 1993; 18:238–44.

[9] Eaton RG, Littler JW. Ligament reconstruction for the painful thumb carpometacarpal joint. J Bone Joint Surg Am 1973;55:1655–66.

[10] Eaton RG, Glickel SZ. Trapeziometacarpal osteoarthritis: staging as a rationale for treatment. Hand Clin 1987;3:455–71.

[11] Swigart CR, Eaton RG, Glickel SZ, et al. Splinting in the treatment of arthritis of the first carpometacarpal joint. J Hand Surg [Am] 1999;24:86–91.

[12] Day CS, Gelberman R, Patel AA, et al. Basal joint osteoarthritis of the thumb: a prospective trial of steroid injection and splinting. J Hand Surg [Am] 2004;29:247–51.

[13] Dell PC, Brushart TM, Smith RJ. Treatment of trapeziometacarpal arthritis: results of resection arthroplasty. J Hand Surg [Am] 1978;3:243–9.

[14] Eaton RG, Lane LB, Littler JW, et al. Ligament reconstruction for the painful thumb carpometacarpal joint: a long-term assessment. J Hand Surg [Am] 1984;61:76–82.

[15] Hobby J, Lyall HA, Meggitt BF. First metacarpal osteotomy for trapeziometacarpal osteoarthritis. J Bone Joint Surg Br 1998;80:508–12.

[16] Tomaino MM. Treatment of Eaton stage I trapeziometacarpal disease with thumb metacarpal extension osteotomy. J Hand Surg [Am] 2000;25:1100–6.

[17] Carroll RE. Arthrodesis of the carpometacarpal joint of the thumb. A review of patients with a long postoperative period. Clin Orthop 1987;220:106–10.

[18] Fulton DB, Stern PJ. Trapeziometacarpal arthrodesis in primary osteoarthritis: a minimum two year follow-up study. J Hand Surg [Am] 2001;26:109–14.

[19] Schwendeman LJ, Stern PJ. Trapeziometacarpal joint fusion. Atlas of the Hand Clinics 1997;2:169–82.

[20] Hanel DP, Condit DP. Thumb carpometacarpal joint fusion with plate and screw fixation. Atlas of the Hand Clinics 1998;3:41–59.

[21] Eaton RG, Littler JW. A study of the basal joint of the thumb. Treatment of its disabilities by fusion. J Bone Joint Surg Am 1969;51:661–8.

[22] Naidu S, Temple JD. Arthritis. In: Beredjiklian PK, Bozentka DJ, editors. Review of hand surgery. Philadelphia: Elsevier; 2004. p. 171–87.

[23] Stark HH, Moore JF, Ashworth CR, et al. Fusion of the first metacarpotrapezial joint for degenerative arthritis. J Bone Joint Surg Am 1977;59:22–6.

[24] Cavallazzi RM, Spreafico G. Trapezio-metacarpal arthrodesis today: why? J Hand Surg [Br] 1986;11:250–4.

[25] Alberts KA, Engkvist O. Arthrodesis of the first carpo-metacarpal joint. Acta Orthop Scand 1989;60:258–60.

[26] Clough DA, Crouch CC, Bennett JB. Failure of trapeziometacarpal arthrodesis with use of the Herbert screw and limited immobilization. J Hand Surg [Am] 1990;15:706–11.

[27] Kvarnes L, Reikeras O. Osteoarthritis of the carpo-metacarpal joint of the thumb. An analysis of operative procedures. J Hand Surg [Br] 1985;10: 117–20.

[28] Hartigan BJ, Stern PJ, Kiefhaber TR. Thumb carpometacarpal osteoarthritis: arthrodesis compared with ligament reconstruction and tendon interposition. J Bone Joint Surg Am 2001;83: 1470–8.

[29] Forseth MJ, Stern PJ. Complications of trapeziometacarpal arthrodesis using plate and screw fixation. J Hand Surg [Am] 2003;28:342–5.

[30] Carroll RE, Hill NA. Arthrodesis of the carpometacarpal joint of the thumb. J Bone Joint Surg Br 1973;55:292–4.

Carpometacarpal Joint Disease: Addressing the Metacarpophalangeal Joint Deformity

Edward J. Armbruster, DO, MA, Virak Tan, MD*

Department of Orthopaedics, Division of Hand and Microvascular Surgery, New Jersey Medical School, University of Medicine and Dentistry of New Jersey, ACC – D1626, 140 Bergen Street, Newark, NJ 07103, USA

Degenerative joint disease occurring at the carpometacarpal (CMC) or basal joint of the thumb has been well studied, and radiographic staging systems have been developed to assist in treatment decision making. The classic deformity that develops in advanced stages of CMC arthrosis is characterized by hyperextension of the thumb metacarpophalangeal (MCP) joint and adduction involving the first web space of the hand (Fig. 1). When taken together, these deformities cause a significant reduction in pinch strength and a diminished ability to grasp large objects, such as the lid of a jar. Several theories have been suggested to account for the adduction deformity, including adductor muscle spasm [1], contracted adductor pollicis muscle belly [2], contracture of overlying fascia [3], and fibrosis and joint stiffness [4]. Although each has been postulated to result in the observed adduction deformity, no singular concept has emerged as causative.

In regard to the observed extension deformity at the MCP joint of the thumb, Landsmeer [5] described the concept of longitudinal collapse progressing in a zigzag fashion along an intercalated axis. In advanced thumb CMC arthrosis, the metacarpal assumes an adducted posture with dorsoradial subluxation of its base on the trapezium. This subluxation is believed to be due to failure of the volar beak ligament [6]. Conventional teaching suggests that the MCP joint assumes an extended moment secondary to this deformity and the pull of extensor pollicis brevis (EPB) (Fig. 2) [7]. Recent studies have called into question these assumptions by noting that the MCP joint bears most of the mechanical stress experienced by the first ray and, as such, the primary deformity (hypermobility progressing to extension) occurs at the MCP joint. CMC subluxation, therefore, would occur secondarily as a result of MCP hypermobility [8]. This approach to understanding intercalated collapse in the thumb ray is a new one and additional studies are required to substantiate these findings.

Addressing the deformity present at the MCP joint of the thumb is paramount in alleviating painful thumb CMC arthrosis and restoring function to the first ray of the hand. One major complication of any CMC reconstruction is failure to recognize and treat the MCP deformity when present, which may result in continued pain and poor outcomes. Additionally, the stability of the ligament reconstruction may become compromised, resulting in recurrence of deformity and longitudinal collapse. It is therefore necessary to give thoughtful attention and careful consideration to the thumb MCP joint when considering treatment options for symptomatic thumb CMC arthrosis.

In examining the patient who has debilitating CMC arthrosis, it is important to note not only symptoms referable to the CMC joint, but also the posture and active and passive ranges of motion of the MCP and interphalangeal joints. Pinch strength, with contralateral comparison, should be noted. Plain radiographs obtained in the anteroposterior, lateral, and oblique planes (for sesamoid evaluation) assist in determining the extent of bony deformity, and facilitate surgical

---

* Corresponding author.

E-mail address: tanvi@umdnj.edu (V. Tan).

doi:10.1016/j.hcl.2008.03.013

hand.theclinics.com

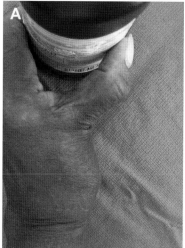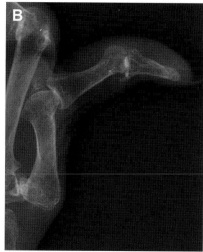

Fig. 1. (A) Patient demonstrating the thumb metacarpal adduction and MCP hyperextension deformities. This patient's ability to grasp an object tightly is severely compromised. (B) Lateral radiograph of the thumb, demonstrating the deformities seen in A. Note dorsoradial subluxation of the base of the first metacarpal.

planning. Specific attention should be directed to assessing the thumb MCP joint for degenerative changes. Such changes influence the surgeon's decision pertaining to any operative intervention

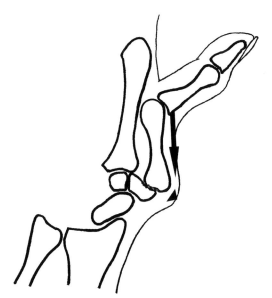

Fig. 2. Forces responsible for the observed adduction and hyperextension deformities. The arrowhead indicates the direction of subluxation of the base of the thumb metacarpal (due to incompetent volar beak ligament). The arrow represents the force vector of the EPB potentiating the MCP hyperextension deformity. A zigzag deformity results, as described by Landsmeer.

that may be required to address the hyperextension/adduction deformity effectively.

Treatment of the MCP hyperextension/adduction deformity is based on physical examination and radiographic findings of degenerative joint disease. In the schema originally outlined by Blank and Feldon [7], the treatment algorithm is determined by the passive flexion of the thumb MCP joint and the presence or absence of degenerative changes. Careful attention to these areas will assist the surgeon in maximizing surgical outcomes.

Metacarpophalangeal joint hyperextension of 0° to 10°

Surgical intervention is not necessary when MCP hyperextension is less than 10°. Often, CMC arthroplasty itself is sufficient to correct any minor deformity. With residual deformity, however, treatment is necessary and is accomplished by postoperative thumb spica casting with the MCP maintained at 20° of flexion [7].

Metacarpophalangeal joint hyperextension of 10° to 20°

Two surgical treatment options, or their combination, exist to address MCP hyperextension of 10° to 20° effectively. By virtue of its insertion on the dorsal aspect of the base of the proximal phalanx, the EPB is a dynamic source of deformity and acts unopposed in extending a hypermobile thumb MCP joint. By redirecting the force vector pull of the EPB to a more radial and proximal location by transferring the insertion to the thumb metacarpal, metacarpal abduction is improved and the extension forces across the joint are diminished [7,9]. Percutaneous pinning of the MCP joint in 25° to 35° of flexion may be performed independently or as an adjunct to EPB transfer. Kirschner wires are maintained for 3 to 4 weeks postoperatively [7].

Kessler [9] described a method of redirecting the EPB tendon while reinforcing the volar capsule of the MCP joint of the thumb. The EPB is released from its musculotendinous junction and routed between the joint capsule and flexor tendon sheath. The tendon is then passed through a bone tunnel drilled through the metacarpal neck, perpendicular to the long axis of the metacarpal. The tendon then crosses itself on the volar aspect of the joint and is sutured to the insertion of the adductor pollicis. In a retrospective study evaluating the efficacy of his procedure, the investigator noted reliable results in terms of pain relief and absence of extension deformity in 7 of 11 patients at an average follow-up of 6.5 years.

Metacarpophalangeal joint hyperextension of 20° to 40°

More aggressive treatment is warranted when MCP extension is between 20° and 40°. If flexion is a minimum of 35° and the MCP joint is congruent and free of arthritis changes, more extensive soft tissue procedures are indicated for the treatment of hypermobility. Capsulodesis of the volar aspect of the MCP joint has been recommended as an effective means of providing a check rein for hyperextension. Sesamoidesis has also been investigated, in addition to capsulodesis. The results of these procedures are encouraging.

In 1957, Zancolli [10] described a technique of volar capsulodesis to correct hyperextension deformity in the fingers of patients who have claw hand due to intrinsic paralysis. Twenty-two years later, he modified his original technique to address the hyperextension deformity seen in the MCP joints of patients who have cerebral palsy. His technique included sesamoidesis not only to correct the hyperextensible joint but also to allow a functional range of motion [11].

Filler and colleagues [12] also performed MCP capsulodesis for hyperextension deformity in children who had cerebral palsy. Their technique uses advancement of the volar plate to the dorsum of the thumb. The investigators reported their experience with 13 thumbs in which initial correction ranged from 20° to 30°. This correction was lost in 2 patients; however, the hyperextension deformity did not recur.

Eaton and Floyd [13] evaluated their results with volar capsulodesis performed in conjunction with basal joint arthroplasty in patients who had collapse deformity of the first ray. Their indication for the procedure was an MCP extension deformity of at least 30°. Instead of using the entire volar capsule, as had been recommended by Zancolli and Filler, their construct used the radial half of the palmar plate, which was advanced proximally over decorticated bone. Traction sutures were brought from the capsule to the dorsum of the metacarpal shaft for fixation. They followed 13 patients for a minimum of 12 months and reported 92% excellent or good results. Pinch strength was reported to be improved by an average of 50%.

Schuurman and Bos [14] reported their findings in the treatment of volar instability of the MCP joint of the thumb with capsulodesis. They used the technique as originally described by Filler [12]. The investigators treated 10 thumbs, with an average follow-up of 15.2 months. They noted that, at last evaluation, all patients had a stable MCP joint, no pain, and no recurrence of hyperextension deformity. The investigators did note, however, that, although the operation is straightforward, it is not to be considered easy because the operative exposure is limited and the local anatomy, challenging.

Tonkin and colleagues [15] reexamined sesamoid arthrodesis for hyperextension of the thumb MCP joint in 1995. The procedures were performed for cerebral palsy or posttraumatic arthropathy, or in conjunction with basal joint arthroplasty. A modification of the Zancolli [11] procedure was used, in which sesamoidesis was combined with capsular advancement and capsulodesis. A total of 42 procedures were reviewed, one half of which were in association with CMC arthroplasty. These 21 patients were followed for an average of 24 months. The investigators found that preoperative MCP hyperextension was decreased from an average of 23° to 4° of flexion postoperatively. No postoperative instability was reported. A total of 4 patients experienced recurrence of hyperextension deformity. The investigators concluded that the procedure was successful in terms of correction of deformity and maintenance of correction.

Additional reports describing techniques to address the MCP hyperextension deformity are limited. In 1981, Eiken [16] proposed a tenodesis, using palmaris longus. Capsulodesis, he believed, was "tricky to perform," and the capsule, already being attenuated, was not considered reliable to resist continued stretch. The transposed palmaris tendon graft acted as a check rein when the thumb was in abduction. In adduction, however, the graft became lax, and hyperextension again became possible. Saadeh and colleagues [17] have recently explored rebalancing the forces across the MCP joint when performing a CMC resection arthroplasty. These researchers describe a method of trapezium excision with resection of the radial half of the trapezoid. No ligament reconstruction is performed. By translating the base of the thumb metacarpal in an ulnar direction, they found that the thumb hyperextension deformity was corrected. In addition, the deforming forces that bring about metacarpal flexion and

adduction are redirected. Fifteen patients were followed for as long as 2 years postoperatively; however, specifics regarding the degree of initial hyperextension deformity, surgical correction of such deformity, and maintenance of deformity, are lacking.

Metacarpophalangeal joint hyperextension of greater than 40°

Arthrodesis is the treatment of choice when thumb MCP hyperextension exceeds 40°, the deformity is not passively correctable, or advanced degenerative changes are noted to affect the articulation. Several techniques have been described to achieve arthrodesis of the MCP joint in 15° to 25° of flexion, neutral valgus/varus, and slight pronation [7]. These techniques include tension banding [18], compression plating [19], lag screw fixation [7], intraosseous wiring [20], or bioabsorbable rods [21]. Regardless of the technique chosen, the goal is to obtain a stable arthrodesis in the desired position to maximize function.

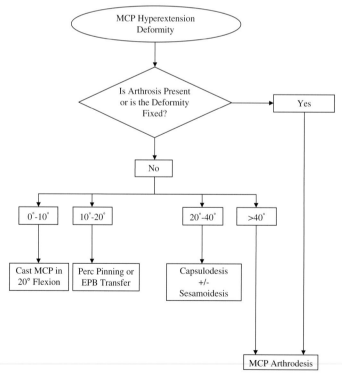

Fig. 3. Algorithm correlating clinical and radiographic findings with treatment recommendations. *Abbreviation:* Perc, percutaneous.

Summary

Successful surgical treatment of basilar thumb arthrosis requires a thorough knowledge of the intercalated longitudinal collapse deformity that occurs with this condition. The arthritic process is initiated by attenuation of the anterior oblique ligament. This attenuation results in capsular laxity, which, when compounded by heterotopic osteophytes, results in dorsoradial subluxation of the thumb metacarpal on the trapezium. With progressive subluxation, the first metacarpal is forced into flexion and adduction. Understanding, recognizing, and effectively addressing the hyperextension deformity is essential to maximize a functional outcome. In evaluating the patient who has symptomatic CMC arthrosis, it is important to note the degree of deformity, passive range of motion, and radiographic findings of joint degeneration. The surgeon may then plan operative intervention accordingly when treating degenerative deformities of the first ray.

An algorithm based on the work of Blank and Feldon (Fig. 3) [7] is provided to correlate clinical and radiographic findings with treatment recommendations. Since the publication of their manuscript in 1997, their treatment outline has not changed significantly; however, several modifications of core techniques have been attempted, with mixed results. Although MCP arthroplasty is an option for the treatment of MCP arthrosis, its role in addressing the hyperextension deformity has not been studied. Regardless, any treatment of the MCP deformity must take into consideration the rebalancing of forces and joint arthrosis. In this light, MCP arthroplasty may represent a future direction in the overall treatment of thumb ray longitudinal collapse deformities.

References

[1] Swanson AB. Disabling arthritis at the base of the thumb: treatment by resection of the trapezium and flexible (silicone) implant arthroplasty. J Bone Joint Surg Am 1972;54:456–71.

[2] Clayton ML. Surgery of the thumb in rheumatoid arthritis. J Bone Joint Surg Am 1962;44:1376–83.

[3] Kessler I. Aetiology management of adduction contracture of the thumb in rheumatoid arthritis. Hand 1973;5:170–4.

[4] Vainio K. Surgery of rheumatoid arthritis. Surg Annu 1974;6:309–35.

[5] Landsmeer JM. The coordination of finger joint motions. J Bone Joint Surg Am 1963;45:1654–62.

[6] Pellegrini VD. Osteoarthritis of the trapeziometacarpal joint: the pathophysiology of articular cartilage degeneration. I. Anatomy and pathology of the aging joint. J Hand Surg [Am] 1991;16(6):967–74.

[7] Blank J, Feldon P. Thumb metacarpophalangeal joint stabilization during carpometacarpal joint surgery. Atlas Hand Clin 1997;2:217–25.

[8] Moulton MJ, Parentis MA, Kelly MJ, et al. Influence of metacarpophalangeal joint position on basal joint-loading in the thumb. J Bone Joint Surg Am 2001;83(5):709–16.

[9] Kessler I. A simplified technique to correct hyperextension deformity of the metacarpophalangeal joint of the thumb. J Bone Joint Surg Am 1979;61(6):903–5.

[10] Zancolli EA. Claw hand caused by paralysis of the intrinsic muscles. A simple procedure for its correction. J Bone Joint Surg Am 1957;39:1076–80.

[11] Zancolli EA. Structural and dynamic bases of hand surgery. 2nd edition. Philadelphia: JB Lippincott; 1979. p. 212.

[12] Filler BC, Stark HH, Boyes JH. Capsulodesis of the metacarpophalangeal joint of the thumb in children with cerebral palsy. J Bone Joint Surg Am 1976;58:667–70.

[13] Eaton RG, Floyd WE III. Thumb metacarpophalangeal capsulodesis: an adjunct procedure to basal joint arthroplasty for collapse deformity of the first ray. J Hand Surg [Am] 1988;13:449–53.

[14] Schuurman AH, Bos KE. Treatment of volar instability of the metacarpophalangeal joint of the thumb by volar capsulodesis. J Bone Joint Surg [Br] 1993;18:346–9.

[15] Tonkin MA, Beard AJ, Kemp SJ, et al. Sigmoid arthrodesis for hyperextension of the thumb metacarpophalangeal joint. J Hand Surg [Am] 1995;20:334–8.

[16] Eiken O. Palmaris longus tenodesis for hyperextension of the thumb metacarpophalangeal joint. Scand J Plast Reconstr Surg 1981;15:149–52.

[17] Saadeh PB, Kazanowski MA, Sharma S, et al. Rebalancing of forces as an adjunct to resection suspension arthroplasty for trapezial arthritis. Ann Plast Surg 2004;52(6):567–70.

[18] Allenda BT, Engelen JC. Tension band arthrodesis in the finger joints. J Hand Surg [Am] 1980;5:269–71.

[19] Wright CS, McMurtry RY. AO arthrodesis in the hand. J Hand Surg [Am] 1983;8:932–5.

[20] Zimmerman NB, Weiland AJ. Ninety-ninety intraosseous wiring for internal fixation of the digital skeleton. Orthopedics 1989;12:99–104.

[21] Voche P, Merle M, Membre H, et al. Bioabsorbable rods and pins for fixation of metacarpophalangeal arthrodesis of the thumb. J Hand Surg [Am] 1995;20:1032–6.

ELSEVIER
SAUNDERS

Hand Clin 24 (2008) 301–306

HAND
CLINICS

Treatment of Scaphotrapezio-Trapezoid Arthritis

Jennifer Moriatis Wolf, MD

Department of Orthopaedics, University of Colorado Denver School of Medicine,
12631 East 17th Avenue, PO Box 6511, Mail Stop B202, Aurora, CO 80045, USA

Although osteoarthritis of the trapeziometa-carpal (TM) joint of the thumb is common, few studies have focused on scaphotrapezio-trapezoid (STT) arthritis. Degenerative arthritis at the articulation of the scaphoid, trapezium, and trapezoid has been described in isolation [1,2] as well as in association with TM arthritis [3]. STT arthritis is often an incidental finding on radiographs [4]. One report showed a radiographic incidence of isolated STT arthritis of 9% [5]. North and Eaton found STT arthritis in 16 of 68 cadaver wrists in a cohort with an average age of 75 years [6]. In an anatomic study of 393 cadaver wrists with an average age of 67 years, Viegas and colleagues [7] showed an average incidence of 20% of wrists with some degree of arthrosis at the STT articulation. In another cadaveric study, 73 wrists with an average age of 84 years showed evidence of STT arthritis in 83% [8].

Although injury to the STT joint alone is rare, arthritis secondary to trauma has been described [9]. One report noted asymptomatic STT arthritis after scaphoid screw placement for fracture through the distal pole of the scaphoid [10]. An alteration in the normal biomechanics of the peri-trapezial joint is thought to be the most common cause of STT arthritis because of the association seen between carpometacarpal and STT arthritis [11,12].

Another theory of etiology is that of chronic wrist instability, specifically based on observed associations between scapholunate instability and STT arthritis. Ferris and colleagues [5] noted an association between STT arthritis and static dorsal intercalated segment instability (DISI) deformity in their radiographic analysis of 697 wrists. More recently, Tay and colleagues [2] evaluated 24 wrists in 16 patients with STT arthritis and DISI deformity. They noted that the scaphoid was extended in these cases rather than flexed as usually seen in DISI and proposed that STT arthritis was a marker for nondissociative carpal instability.

Anatomy

The scaphoid bridges the proximal and distal rows of the carpus on its radial side. The scaphoid has articulations with the scaphoid fossa of the distal radius, the lunate, the capitate, the trapezium, and the trapezoid (Fig. 1). Moritomo and colleagues [13] described the interfacet ridge of the distal scaphoid, which is aligned from radiodorsal to ulnar-volar and was present in 81% of cadaver wrists studied. Superior to and lateral to the scaphoid, the trapezium articulates with the scaphoid and the base of the first metacarpal via its unique saddle-shaped joint surface. Medially, the trapezoid articulates with the trapezium and the scaphoid as well as the capitate, and also provides articulation for the base of the second metacarpal.

The major ligaments of the STT articulation include the trapeziotrapezoid, the trapezoid-capitate, and the STT ligaments [14]. The trapeziotrapezoid ligament has volar and dorsal components and spans the length of the joint between the trapezium and trapezoid. The thick, deep, trapezocapitate ligament runs at an angle in a notch between the trapezoid and capitate to insert on the capitate waist. Volarly, the STT ligament originates from the radial and ulnar sides of the scaphoid and then divides into two bands. The scaphotrapezial band connects the scaphoid and

E-mail address: jennifer.wolf@uchsc.edu

0749-0712/08/$ - see front matter © 2008 Elsevier Inc. All rights reserved.
doi:10.1016/j.hcl.2008.03.002

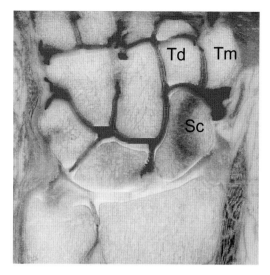

Fig. 1. Coronal view of the hand. The STT joint is seen. Sc, scaphoid; Tm, trapezium; Td, trapezoid. (*Courtesy of the Visible Hand, Center for Human Simulation, University of Colorado Denver, Aurora, CO; with permission.*)

trapezium, with fibers forming a V-shape. The scaphotrapezoid band connects the ulnar aspect of the scaphoid to the volar trapezoid [14,15].

Clinical presentation

Because STT and TM arthritis are often coexistent, patients often present with complaints of basilar thumb pain. Tomaino and colleagues [12] noted that in patients with arthrosis of both joints, they were unable to differentiate between the two on physical examination, including use of the crank and grind tests. In isolated STT arthritis, pain is often localized as more medial, within the thenar eminence, and is noted as a deep aching pain not necessarily associated with thumb motion.

Most clinical studies of STT arthritis describe its incidence in association with TM arthritis. Presumably, the age at presentation is likely similar, with STT arthritis occurring more frequently in postmenopausal women, with a peak in incidence at 50 to 70 years of age [3]. Tay's radiographic study supports this, with a group of 16 patients with findings of STT arthritis, predominantly females, with an average age of 60 years [2].

Imaging

Radiographs of the base of the thumb taken in three planes are standard for visualization of the STT and TM joints (Fig. 2). Additionally, a stress view of the TM joint can be used to show the degree of laxity of the basilar thumb joint [3]. Recently, Wollstein and colleagues [16] described a specific STT view for optimal visualization of these joints. This view is performed with the patient standing, with the wrist in maximal extension and ulnar deviation with the hand an inch above the x-ray cassette, and with the beam directed perpendicular to approximately 2.5 cm medial to the base of the thumb TM joint. Findings of narrowing between the scaphoid and trapezoid, or trapezium, as well as the presence of osteophytes indicate the presence of STT arthritis (Fig. 2).

Several studies have noted that radiographs underestimate the degree and severity of STT arthritis. Glickel and colleagues [17] noted that the findings at surgery matched the radiographic evaluation of the STT joint approximately 66% of the time. More recently, Brown and colleagues [11] noted a correlation between radiographs and visual STT arthritis in only 39% of cadaveric specimens.

Conservative treatment of scaphotrapezio-trapezoid arthritis

Nonoperative therapy for STT arthritis is recommended as the initial treatment course, similar to management of TM arthritis. Activity modification, rest, the use of splints, and injection of the affected joint or joints can be helpful [3]. Activity modification consists of avoiding forceful pinch and using adaptive equipment such as jar top openers. Splinting can consist of either long or short thumb opponens splints or both; studies have shown that short opponens splints are preferred by patients [18]. Often, patients find it most helpful to wear these splints at night to rest the joint.

Corticosteroid injections have not been studied specifically for STT arthritis. Their use in TM arthritis has been evaluated in several reports. In patients with early stage arthritis, corticosteroid injection has been shown to give good pain relief for up to 2 years when combined with splinting [19]. Another study showed only short-term effects of corticosteroid injections, with no impact on pain scores or function past 1 month [20].

Operative treatment of scaphotrapezio-trapezoid arthritis

Arthrodesis

Although the technique of STT fusion was described in the mid-1900s [21], Watson and

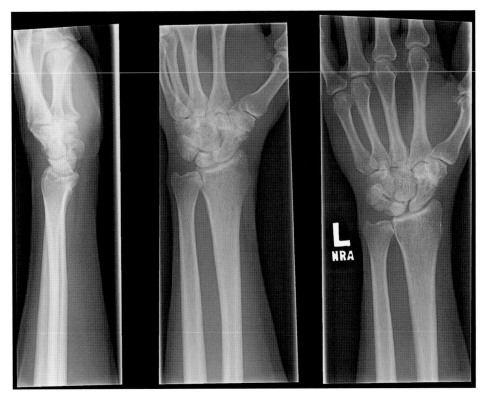

Fig. 2. Radiograph of the carpometacarpal and STT joint in three planes. Note the narrowing and osteophyte formation of the STT joint.

Hempton [22] produced one of the earliest comprehensive reports on the operative treatment of STT arthritis in 1980. This arthrodesis was reported to "leave the wrist strong with minimal loss of motion." Since that report, STT fusion has been recommended for STT arthritis, scapholunate instability, and advanced stages of Kienbock's disease [23–27]. The procedure is generally performed through a dorsal radial incision, either transverse or oblique. The joint surfaces are decorticated and packed with graft from the iliac crest or distal radius. Fixation of the fusion mass is classically achieved using Kirschner wires which are later removed [28]. Alternative methods of fixation include small limited fusion plates (Fig. 3) or headless screw fixation.

In Watson's series, triscaphe fusion was performed using three 0.045-in Kirschner wires in 13 patients, 7 of whom had degenerative changes of the STT joint. Outcomes were good overall, with a flexion-extension arc of motion of 104 degrees and stated pain relief. There was one nonunion and three cases of shoulder-hand syndrome (similar to chronic regional pain syndrome) [22].

Frykman and colleagues [29] reported their 2-year results of STT arthrodesis performed in patients with scaphoid instability (rotatory subluxation) and STT arthritis, without segregation of the results by indication. They noted loss of motion of an average of 36 degrees of flexion and 41 degrees of extension. Five of 17 hands went on to nonunion of the STT joint, with four requiring reoperation. Two other cases required total wrist fusion due to persistent pain despite solid bony union. Another author performed five STT arthrodeses for degenerative joint disease, with an average of 3 years of follow-up, and reported fair patient satisfaction with one nonunion requiring revision [23].

Studies with longer follow-up have shown more mixed outcomes. Fortin and Louis [24] presented a series of 14 patients who underwent STT fusion for isolated arthritis or chronic scapholunate instability, with an average follow-up over 5 years. Ten of the 14 patients had radiographic

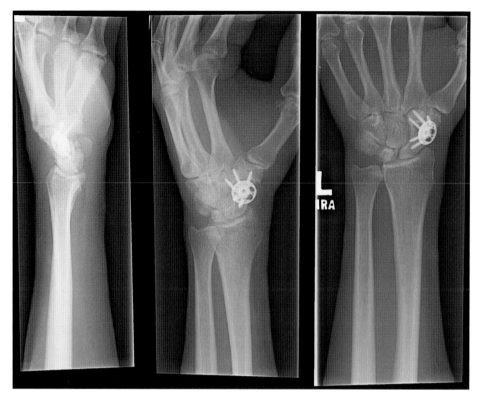

Fig. 3. Use of a small limited fusion plate for STT arthrodesis. (*Courtesy of* Francis Scott, MD, Aurora, CO.)

evidence of arthrosis at the radiocarpal or TM joints, and three went on to nonunion. They noted the importance of aligning the scaphoid in a normal orientation but noted that, even with a technically well-positioned arthrodesis, patients had significant functional limitations. More recently, Minami and colleagues [30] reported the 7-year follow-up of a cohort of 30 patients who underwent STT arthrodesis for Kienböck's disease, STT arthrosis, and traumatic dislocation of the trapezium. Subjectively, 26 of 30 patients were satisfied, and grip strength significantly improved ($P < .05$). There were no nonunions, but 27% experienced complications postoperatively, including radioscaphoid and TM arthritis in seven patients.

Other procedures

Since fusion has been the primary procedure described, there is limited literature on other options for isolated STT arthritis. In the review of STT arthritis by Crosby and colleagues [23], they described fibrous arthroplasty, interposition arthroplasty, and trapezial replacement arthroplasty as options. Fibrous arthroplasty involved excision of 3 to 4 mm of the distal articulation of the scaphoid, with interposition of a portion of the flexor carpi radialis tendon. Interposition arthroplasty similarly removed a portion of the scaphoid but replaced it with a stemmed Kessler implant originally intended for use at the TM joint. Trapezial arthroplasty was also performed with a silicone trapezial implant. Crosby also described trapezial excision alone in one patient, who required later scaphometacarpal fusion for painful adduction and flexion contracture. The use of STT fusion was thought to offer superior pain relief and strength when compared with these procedures and was advocated by this group.

When STT arthrosis is seen in conjunction with TM arthritis, excision of the proximal trapezoid in combination with trapezial excision has been advocated. Irwin and colleagues [31] suggested that residual STT arthrosis was a potential source of pain after successful surgery for TM arthritis. Tomaino and colleagues [12] reported the outcomes in 23 patients who underwent excision of the proximal 2 mm of trapezoid when joint destruction was noted intraoperatively. When grip and pinch strength was compared with that in a group of patients who underwent only excision of the trapezium as part of a standard ligament reconstruction and tendon interposition procedure, there was no significant difference between the groups.

Complications

Nonunion

Nonunion of the fusion mass has been reported in multiple studies as a complication of STT arthrodesis. In patients, Watson and colleagues [32] reported that nonunion was the most common complication, occurring in 36 patients (4%). Another study in Sweden noted an incidence of five nonunions in 17 hands (29%) treated with STT arthrodesis [29]. McAuliffe and colleagues [33] noted a similar rate of nonunion, with 6 of 25 hands in their series failing to fuse. Fortin and Lewis reported nonunion in 3 of 19 (16%) patients in their series of STT arthrosis.

Nerve injury or irritation and reflex sympathetic dystrophy

One study noted that three patients underwent a total of seven surgeries after STT arthrodesis to treat neuritis or compression of the radial nerve [33]. Another report noted transient irritation of the superficial radial nerve in 2 of 84 cases of STT arthrodesis [26].

In Watson's large series of 800 cases of STT arthrodesis, reflex sympathetic dystrophy occurred in 29 patients (3.6%) These patients were reported to have been treated with a standard management program, but no further outcome of this complication was provided [32]. This study also noted superficial radial neuromas in situ in seven patients, who presumably required surgical treatment.

Radial styloid impingement

Rogers and Watson [34] originally reported the complication of impaction of the scaphoid fusion mass against the radial styloid after STT arthrodesis. They noted this complication in 31 of 93 STT fusions, with a higher incidence in patients who were initially surgically treated for rotatory subluxation of the scaphoid. The patients' pain and impingement resolved with partial radial styloidectomy. This complication was also noted by Kleinman [27] in his 10-year review of STT arthrodesis performed for scapholunate instability

and was managed in two patients by radial styloidectomy.

Secondary arthrosis of other wrist joints

In a study with an average 5-year follow-up (range, 26–96 months), Fortin and Louis [24] noted the development of progressive arthrosis of the radiocarpal and TM joints after STT fusion. They noted radiocarpal degeneration in 6 of 19 patients (32%) and TM arthrosis in four patients (21%). Three of these ten patients went on to further surgery including carpometacarpal arthroplasty and radiocarpal fusion.

Kleinman and Carroll [27] also noted progressive radiocarpal arthrosis in 19% of their series of STT fusion performed for scapholunate instability. Four patients went on to radiocarpal arthrodesis, and two underwent total wrist arthroplasty. This arthritic change occurred in cases in which the scaphoid was malaligned in creation of the fusion mass.

Summary

STT arthritis is often coexistent with TM arthritis but is also seen as an isolated arthrosis of the STT joint. Patients present with deep basilar thumb pain and difficulty with pinch and grasp, similar to TM arthritis. Specific imaging views may be helpful in evaluation of the STT joint.

Conservative treatment consists of activity modification, splinting, and corticosteroid injections. The main operative treatment is arthrodesis of the STT joint, although trapeziectomy, soft tissue interposition, and implant replacement have been described. Complications include nonunion (most common), superficial radial nerve injury, and arthrosis at pericarpal joints.

References

[1] Wadhwani A, Carey J, Propeck T, et al. Isolated scaphotrapeziotrapezoid osteoarthritis: a possible radiographic marker of chronic scapholunate ligament disruption. Clin Radiol 1998;53(5):376–8.
[2] Tay SC, Moran SL, Shin AY, et al. The clinical implications of scaphotrapezium-trapezoidal arthritis with associated carpal instability. J Hand Surg [Am] 2007;32(1):47–54.
[3] Dias R, Chandrasenan J, Rajaratnam V, et al. Basal thumb arthritis. Postgrad Med J 2007;83(975):40–3.
[4] Watson HK, Ryu J. Evolution of arthritis of the wrist. Clin Orthop Relat Res 1986;202:57–67.

[5] Ferris BD, Dunnett W, Lavelle JR. An association between scaphotrapezio-trapezoid osteoarthritis and static dorsal intercalated segment instability. J Hand Surg [Br] 1994;19(3):338–9.

[6] North ER, Eaton RG. Degenerative joint disease of the trapezium: a comparative radiographic and anatomic study. J Hand Surg [Am] 1983;8(2):160–6.

[7] Kleinman WB, Carroll CT. Scapho-trapezio-trapezoid arthrodesis for treatment of chronic static and dynamic scapholunate instability: a 10-year perspective on pitfalls and complications. J Hand Surg [Am] 1990;15:408–14.

[8] Bhatia A, Pisoh T, Touam C, et al. Incidence and distribution of scaphotrapezotrapezoidal arthritis in 73 fresh cadaveric wrists. Ann Chir Main Memb Super 1996;15(4):220–5.

[9] Sicre G, Laulan J, Rouleau B. Scaphotrapeziotrapezoid osteoarthritis after scaphotrapezial ligament injury. J Hand Surg [Br] 1997;22(2):189–90.

[10] Saeden B, Tornkvist H, Ponzer S, et al. Fracture of the carpal scaphoid: a prospective, randomised 12-year follow-up comparing operative and conservative treatment. J Bone Joint Surg Br 2001;83(2):230–4.

[11] Brown GD III, Roh MS, Strauch RJ, et al. Radiography and visual pathology of the osteoarthritic scaphotrapezio-trapezoidal joint, and its relationship to trapeziometacarpal osteoarthritis. J Hand Surg [Am] 2003;28(5):739–43.

[12] Tomaino MM, Vogt M, Weiser R. Scaphotrapezoid arthritis: prevalence in thumbs undergoing trapezium excision arthroplasty and efficacy of proximal trapezoid excision. J Hand Surg [Am] 1999;24(6):1220–4.

[13] Moritomo H, Viegas SF, Nakamura K, et al. The scaphotrapezio-trapezoidal joint. Part 1. An anatomic and radiographic study. J Hand Surg [Am] 2000;25(5):899–910.

[14] Berger RA. The anatomy of the ligaments of the wrist and distal radioulnar joints. Clin Orthop Relat Res 2001;(383):32–40.

[15] Berger RA. The ligaments of the wrist: a current overview of anatomy with considerations of their potential functions. Hand Clin 1997;13(1):63–82.

[16] Wollstein R, Wandzy N, Mastella DJ, et al. A radiographic view of the scaphotrapezium-trapezoid joint. J Hand Surg [Am] 2005;30(6):1161–3.

[17] Glickel SZ, Kornstein AN, Eaton RG. Long-term follow-up of trapeziometacarpal arthroplasty with coexisting scaphotrapezial disease. J Hand Surg [Am] 1992;17(4):612–20.

[18] Weiss S, LaStayo P, Mills A, et al. Prospective analysis of splinting the first carpometacarpal joint: an objective, subjective, and radiographic assessment. J Hand Ther 2000;13(3):218–26.

[19] Day CS, Gelberman R, Patel AA, et al. Basal joint osteoarthritis of the thumb: a prospective trial of steroid injection and splinting. J Hand Surg [Am] 2004;29(2):247–51.

[20] Meenagh GK, Patton J, Kynes C, et al. A randomised controlled trial of intra-articular corticosteroid injection of the carpometacarpal joint of the thumb in osteoarthritis. Ann Rheum Dis 2004;63(10):1260–3.

[21] Peterson HA, Lipscomb PR. Intercarpal arthrodesis. Arch Surg 1967;95(1):127–34.

[22] Watson HK, Hempton RF. Limited wrist arthrodeses. I. The triscaphoid joint. J Hand Surg [Am] 1980;5(4):320–7.

[23] Crosby EB, Linscheid RL, Dobyns JH. Scaphotrapezial trapezoidal arthrosis. J Hand Surg [Am] 1978;3(3):223–34.

[24] Fortin PT, Louis DS. Long-term follow-up of scaphoid-trapezium-trapezoid arthrodesis. J Hand Surg [Am] 1993;18(4):675–81.

[25] Ishikawa J, Iwasaki N, Minami A. Influence of distal radioulnar joint subluxation on restricted forearm rotation after distal radius fracture. J Hand Surg [Am] 2005;30(6):1178–84.

[26] Meier R, van Griensven M, Krimmer H. Scaphotrapeziotrapezoid (STT)-arthrodesis in Kienbock's disease. J Hand Surg [Br] 2004;29(6):580–4.

[27] Kleinman WB. Long-term study of chronic scapholunate instability treated by scapho-trapezio-trapezoid arthrodesis. J Hand Surg [Am] 1989;14(3):429–45.

[28] Wollstein R, Watson HK. Scaphotrapeziotrapezoid arthrodesis for arthritis. Hand Clin 2005;21(4):539–43.

[29] Frykman EB, Af Ekenstam F, Wadin K. Triscaphoid arthrodesis and its complications. J Hand Surg [Am] 1988;13(6):844–9.

[30] Minami A, Kato H, Suenaga N, et al. Scaphotrapeziotrapezoid fusion: long-term follow-up study. J Orthop Sci 2003;8(3):319–22.

[31] Irwin AS, Maffulli N, Chesney RB. Scapho-trapezoid arthritis: a cause of residual pain after arthroplasty of the trapezio-metacarpal joint. J Hand Surg [Br] 1995;20(3):346–52.

[32] Watson HK, Wollstein R, Joseph E, et al. Scaphotrapeziotrapezoid arthrodesis: a follow-up study. J Hand Surg [Am] 2003;28(3):397–404.

[33] McAuliffe JA, Dell PC, Jaffe R. Complications of intercarpal arthrodesis. J Hand Surg [Am] 1993;18(6):1121–8.

[34] Rogers WD, Watson HK. Radial styloid impingement after triscaphe arthrodesis. J Hand Surg [Am] 1989;14(2 Pt 1):297–301.

The Rheumatoid Thumb

Aron T. Chacko, BS[a], Tamara D. Rozental, MD[b],*

[a]*Department of Orthopaedic Surgery, Beth Israel Deaconess Medical Center, Harvard Medical School,*
330 Brookline Avenue, Stoneman 10, Boston, MA 02215, USA
[b]*Harvard Medical School, Beth Israel Deaconess Medical Center, 330 Brookline Avenue,*
Stoneman 10, Boston, MA 02215, USA

Rheumatoid arthritis is a systemic disease affecting 0.3% to 1.5% of the population of the United States. It is three times more likely to involve women than men [1]. By limiting grip and pinch strength, rheumatoid arthritis of the thumb severely impairs the activities of daily living [2].

Anatomy and pathophysiology

The pathophysiology of rheumatoid arthritis involves synovial proliferation with invasion of periarticular structures and articular cartilage. As the disease progresses, the synovial pannus grows, and ligaments and tendons become incompetent, which leads to the loss of bone stock and malalignment and hindering of thumb function.

In 1968, Nalebuff [3] devised a classification system for thumb deformities in rheumatoid arthritis. This classification takes into account the degree of severity of the imbalance and the involvement of adjacent structures. Thumb deformities are now classified from type I to type VI.

The type I, or boutonniere, deformity is the most common. It presents with flexion at the metacarpophalangeal joint (MP) and hyperextension at the interphalangeal (IP) joint (Figs. 1 and 2). Laxity of the dorsal capsule results from proliferative synovitis around the MP joint, in turn allowing volar and ulnar subluxation of the

Modified with permission. Significant portions of this article are directly reprinted from the following: ©2007 American Academy of Orthopedic Surgeons. Reprinted from the *Journal of the American Academy of Orthopedic Surgeons*, Volume 15(2). pp.118–125; with permission.
* Corresponding author.
E-mail address: trozenta@bidmc.harvard.edu (T.D. Rozental).

extensor pollicis longus (EPL) tendon, which results in MP joint flexion and weakening of active extension. Subluxation of the EPL tendon then causes IP joint hyperextension and adduction of the first metacarpal. With progression of the disease, the deformity becomes fixed and can no longer be corrected passively. A similar deformity can be seen in patients who have a flexor pollicis longus tendon rupture or attenuation of the volar capsule. In these cases, IP hyperextension occurs and results in MP joint flexion.

The type II deformity also presents with MP flexion, IP hyperextension, and metacarpal adduction but it involves the carpometacarpal joint (CMC). The second most common deformity is the type III, or swan-neck, deformity. In this case, MP hyperextension, IP flexion, and metacarpal adduction (Figs. 3 and 4) result from proliferative synovitis at the CMC joint. Volar plate laxity and dorsal and radial shift of the metacarpal base contribute to an imbalance of the extensor forces.

Three additional patterns of thumb involvement were added to the original Nalebuff classification [4]. The type IV deformity is characterized by lateral instability of the MP joint secondary to attenuation of the ulnar collateral ligament. Type V deformities are similar to type III swan-neck deformities, but attenuation of the volar plate is the initiating factor. In these patients, the CMC joint is usually not involved. Finally, loss of bone stock and skeletal collapse characterize type VI deformities arthritis mutilans (Fig. 5).

Clinical evaluation and conservative treatment

Patients typically present with one of four stages of thumb involvement. In stage 1, synovitis has

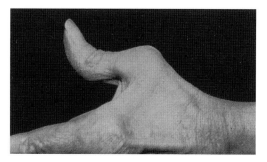

Fig. 1. Type I boutonnière deformity with MP joint flexion and IP joint hyperextension. (*From* Stein AB, Terrono AL. The rheumatoid thumb. Hand Clin 1996;12(3):541–50; with permission.)

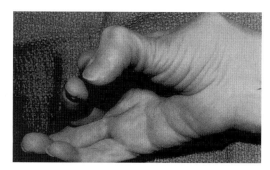

Fig. 3. Type III swan-neck deformity with hyperextension of the MP joint and IP joint flexion. (*From* Stein AB, Terrono AL. The rheumatoid thumb. Hand Clin 1996;12(3):541–50; with permission.)

been present for less than 6 months and responds to conservative medical therapy. In stage 2, synovitis has been present for much longer than 6 months and synovectomy may be performed. Stage 3 is used to classify boutonniere and swan-neck deformities, often treated with reconstructive surgery. Salvage procedures, however, are required to treat arthritis mutilans, classified as stage 4 [5].

Oral medication

Nonsteroidal anti-inflammatories are often the first-line drugs for treating patients in stage 1 of the disease. Disease-modifying antirheumatic

drugs (DMARDs) such as gold, antimalarials, penicillamine, and methotrexate can be added subsequently. DMARDs prevent the continued destruction of the joint but do not treat the inflammation associated with the disease. Cytotoxic drugs (systemic steroids, azathioprine, or cyclosporine) are also used in refractory cases.

Biologic response modifiers, or biologic agents, are gaining popularity. These agents target specific areas in the immune system and slow the progression of disease. Adalimumab, anakinra, etanercept, rituximab, and infliximab are examples of biologic agents that can be used alone or in conjunction with other medications [6].

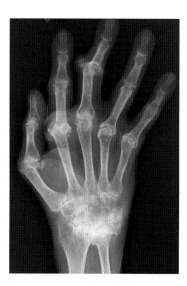

Fig. 2. Posteroanterior radiograph of a type I deformity. Note the degenerative changes most pronounced at the MP joint. (*From* Rozental TD. Reconstruction of the rheumatoid thumb. J Am Acad Orthop Surg 2007;15:118–25; with permission.)

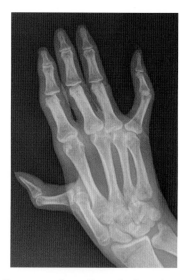

Fig. 4. Posteroanterior radiograph of an advanced type III deformity with subluxation at the CMC and MP joints. (*From* Rozental TD. Reconstruction of the rheumatoid thumb. J Am Acad Orthop Surg 2007;15:118–25; with permission.)

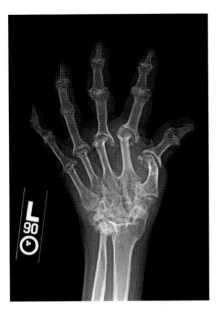

Fig. 5. Anteroposterior radiograph of a patient who has type VI deformity (arthritis mutilans). (*From* Rozental TD. Reconstruction of the rheumatoid thumb. J Am Acad Orthop Surg 2007;15:118–25; with permission.)

Steroid injections

Intra-articular corticosteroids are commonly used in the treatment of early disease. These are most helpful for painful CMC and MP joints. Although no studies have identified an "ideal" steroid preparation, most physicians combine a local anesthetic with 40 mg of methylprednisolone or triamcinolone. Complications with injections are rare [7] but include steroid arthropathy, tendon rupture, avascular necrosis, infection, post-injection flare, and hypersensitivity reactions.

Splinting and occupational therapy

Through immobilization and reduction of synovitis and inflammation, splints are effective in treating painful joints. They can also help maintain joints in alignment and prevent contractures [8]. In more advanced cases, splinting can provide stability and improve overall hand function in performing the activities of daily living. Instruction in activity modification and joint protection is also beneficial; hand-strengthening exercises in particular have been shown to be effective in improving the functional ability of the limb [9,10].

Surgical treatment

Once patients progress to stage 3 of the disease, thumb deformities are often best treated surgically. When determining the optimal operation, the surgeon must take into account involvement of the CMC, MP, and IP joints. A thorough examination of the entire upper extremity should also identify concomitant shoulder or elbow involvement, which may best be addressed first.

Synovectomy

Synovectomy is beneficial in the early stages of disease, before bony destruction is visible on plain radiographs. It is usually indicated in patients who have had MP joint swelling refractory to medical therapy for more than 6 months, or in those who have continued progression of disease. Typically, synovectomy does not alter the progression of the disease, with inflammation returning in up to 15% of patients [11]. Rather, synovectomy is meant to reduce pain and inflammation, thereby improving patients' symptoms.

Concomitant shortening of the extensor mechanism by rerouting the EPL to the dorsal capsule is often performed to provide additional extensor strength [12]. Unfortunately, deformity recurrence is seen in up to 64% of cases [13] and has been attributed to progressive attenuation of the new tendon insertion. The technique has now been modified so that the EPL tendon is inserted directly into bone. Reported results suggest better long-term outcomes and improved extensor strength [14,15].

A second problem noted following EPL rerouting is the inability in certain patients to extend the distal phalanx actively [16]. MP and IP joint range of motion often have an inverse relationship; with improvement in MP range of motion, patients often lose extension at the IP joint. Insertion of the extensor pollicis brevis tendon at the base of the proximal phalanx with extensor hood reconstruction can be performed to address this issue [17].

Capsulodesis

Capsulodesis is used in patients who have a type V deformity secondary to volar plate instability. This procedure can be performed by strengthening the capsule and transposing the extensor pollicis brevis tendon [18] or by suturing the radial aspect of the volar plate to the dorsal aspect of the thumb [19]. A 1993 review of capsule applications showed no cases of recurrent instability in 10 patients treated with the procedure [20].

Tendon repair

Flexion and extension imbalances often result from direct tendon rupture. The causes of tendon ruptures can be traced to synovial infiltration, ischemia (particularly at the distal extensor retinaculum), or erosions over bony prominences.

Extensor pollicis longus rupture

Dorsal tenosynovitis is the most common site of inflammation around the wrist and it presents with dorsal swelling and crepitation. The EPL tendon is most often ruptured as it wraps around Lister's tubercle [21].

Spontaneous ruptures of the EPL tendon may present with a flexion deformity at the IP joint. Although patients may be able to extend the IP joint through the intrinsic musculature, they cannot hyperextend it. In cases of acute tendon rupture, a primary repair may be attempted. Once tendon retraction or loss occurs, however, end-to-end repairs are difficult to perform and tendon transfers become the procedure of choice. The most commonly used tendon procedure involves transferring the extensor indicis proprius to the ruptured EPL. Alternatively, the extensor carpi radialis longus can be used. The authors prefer the extensor indicis proprius because it can be taken without compromising index finger function or wrist radial extension [22,23]. Results with this procedure are encouraging; although patients may have a residual extension lag in the thumb and index, good grip force and dexterity are often obtained [16]. Alternatively, a bridge tendon graft can be used for repair [24]. Finally, patients who have significant bony destruction at the IP joint are best treated with joint arthrodesis.

Flexor pollicis longus rupture

Flexor pollicis longus ruptures are usually secondary to attrition around the scaphoid bone in the carpal tunnel and are referred to as a Mannerfelt lesion [25]. Patients typically present with an acute loss of flexion at the IP joint of the thumb. It is essential to treat these patients with a thorough tenosynovectomy and debridement of any bony prominences. The tendon repair is usually accomplished with a bridge tendon graft or by transfer of the ring finger flexor digitorum superficialis tendon. Results of flexor pollicis longus rupture repair are less favorable than those reported for extensor tendon repair [26].

Replacement arthroplasty

Metacarpophalangeal joint

MP joint arthroplasty is primarily indicated in patients who have severe destruction of the articular surfaces with preserved ligamentous stability. A common indication for MP arthroplasty is a patient who has a boutonniere deformity with a stable MP joint and severe IP joint disease. In these cases, MP arthroplasty is often combined with an IP fusion. MP arthroplasty should not be performed in cases that involve severe hyperextension deformities.

The operative technique consists of splitting the extensor hood and detaching the extensor pollicis brevis from the base of the proximal phalanx. The metacarpal head is resected and the medullary canals of the phalanx and metacarpal are reamed to accept the implants. After implantation, the extensor pollicis brevis tendon is reattached, and the extensor hood repaired. A K-wire may be used to hold the joint in extension during the procedure, and it can subsequently act as an internal splint.

In their original series, Swanson and Herndon [27] reported good-to-excellent results in 42 out of 44 thumbs at 2.5 to 6 years' follow-up. Since then, Terrono and colleagues [23] and Figgie and colleagues [28] have reported successful results with this procedure.

Other implant designs include the Flatt implant, introduced in 1972 [29], and the Steffe cemented implant, described in 1981. Flatt and Steffe implants (initially reported by Blair and colleagues) [30] generated good results but have since been plagued by reports of prosthetic loosening. A recent series of 54 primary arthroplasties with Steffe implants, however, found 93% implant survivorship at 5 years and 89% at 10 years after surgery [31]. Complications encountered following MP joint arthroplasty include implant fracture and infection. Prosthetic fractures complicated 11% of Swanson's reported cases (much lower than prosthetic fractures after finger MP arthroplasty, which were around 26%). Infection rates for Swanson implants are low, ranging from 0.6% to 3% [32]. Silicone synovitis is an uncommon complication following thumb MP arthroplasty, with few reports in the current literature.

MP arthroplasty is thus recommended for patients who have well preserved collateral ligaments despite severe disease. It is best suited for the low-demand patient who has intact proximal and distal joints.

Carpometacarpal joint

CMC replacement arthroplasty can range from partial or complete trapezial implants, to trapezial resection or resurfacing techniques [33].

Initial efforts focused on silicone trapezial arthroplasty and resulted in stable, pain-free thumbs. Long-term results, however, have demonstrated multiple long-term complications, including silicone synovitis and implant subluxation [34–36]. Follow-up studies have shown a 74% incidence of metacarpal cysts and a 56% incidence of scaphoid involvement [37], and implant subluxation has been reported to be as high as 19% [38]. Eaton [39] incorporated a tendon strip for implant stabilization and described a 10% rate of subluxation and dislocation. Problems with synovitis and implant subluxation have led to the development of alternative arthroplasty techniques. The Niebauer silastic design incorporates a polyethylene mesh to allow for bony ingrowth. Despite good short-term results [40], a 9-year follow-up series revealed a high incidence of subluxation [41]. Several titanium implants have become available, but few long-term results have been published to date. A new ceramic interpositional device has recently been introduced to the market, with disappointing results [42].

Total arthroplasty of the thumb CMC joint, replacing metacarpal and trapezial surfaces, has also been attempted, with limited success. Although biomechanical cadaveric studies have shown kinematics and stability similar to the native thumb [43], clinical results have been disappointing. In particular, implant dislocation has been of concern, with failure rates approaching 40% [44].

Interpositional arthroplasty

Trapezial resection suspension arthroplasty procedures are currently the procedures of choice in the treatment of rheumatoid arthritis involving the CMC joint. Initially described in patients who had osteoarthritis, multiple techniques are now available. These techniques range from simple trapezium excision to techniques of tendon interpositional arthroplasty using flexor carpi radialis, palmaris longus, or abductor pollicis longus tendons. The long-term results of these procedures are equivalent, with up to 95% rated as excellent (Fig. 6) [45–50]. The operative

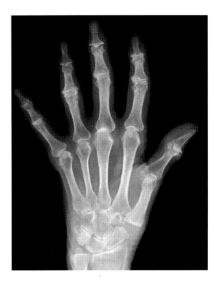

Fig. 6. Posteroanterior radiograph of a hand 2 years after a trapezium resection was done for CMC joint disease. There has been minimal subluxation of the thumb metacarpal, and the patient maintained an excellent functional outcome. (*From* Rozental TD. Reconstruction of the rheumatoid thumb. J Am Acad Orthop Surg 2007;15:118–25; with permission.)

techniques for these individual procedures are described elsewhere in this issue. With most of the literature focusing on osteoarthritis, few follow-up data are currently available for CMC interpositional arthroplasties in patients who have rheumatoid arthritis.

Arthrodesis

Interphalangeal joint

IP joint arthrodesis provides good pain relief and restoration of function in patients who have advanced joint destruction, particularly when the CMC and MCP joints are spared. IP joints are typically fused in neutral alignment or in slight flexion to facilitate pinch.

Arthrodesis methods vary widely and include fixation with K-wires, headless compression screws, and external devices [51,52]. The authors prefer fixation with a headless screw because it allows minimal splinting and early mobilization (Fig. 7) [53]. In most cases, however, good bony fusion has been reported, regardless of fixation method [54]. In the most extreme cases of bony erosion, bone grafting can be a useful adjuvant for enhancing fusion rates.

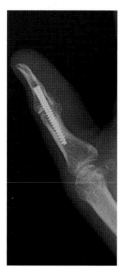

Fig. 7. Lateral radiograph of a thumb IP fusion with a headless compression screw. (*From* Rozental TD. Reconstruction of the rheumatoid thumb. J Am Acad Orthop Surg 2007;15:118–25; with permission.)

Metacarpophalangeal joint

Arthrodesis has been, and continues to be, the gold standard for treatment of MP joint disease. In particular, it is preferred for patients whose adjacent CMC and IP joints are intact. The position for fusion recommended for preservation of pinch function consists of 15 degrees of flexion, 5 degrees of abduction, and 20 degrees of pronation. The operation can be performed with a chevron osteotomy or with a "cup-and-cone" method of decortication. Methods of fixation are varied and include crossed K-wires, interosseous wiring, tension-band techniques, and headless compression or cannulated screws.

Fusion rates are typically good and range from 80% to 100%. Stanley and colleagues [55] reviewed 42 cases of MP arthrodesis and judged 83% of operations to be successful, with 7 cases of pain or instability at the site of fusion and 2 cases of EPL rupture. A 1990 review reported a 13% rate of IP instability and no nonunions [24]. No patient required revision procedure 5 years after surgery. Bone grafting is an important tool in patients who have the severe pencil-in-cup deformities seen in arthritis mutilans [56]. These arthrodeses often require prolonged immobilization, for up to 5 months.

The major disadvantages of MP joint arthrodesis include loss of precision mobility and increased stress placed on adjacent joints, resulting in progression of disease at the CMC and IP articulations [35]. Despite these shortcomings, the authors continue to use MP joint arthrodesis as the mainstay of treatment of moderate-type deformities in active patients requiring strong and stable thumbs.

Carpometacarpal joint

Arthrodesis of the CMC joint is uncommon. It is typically recommended for young patients who have isolated CMC trapeziometacarpal disease. Although studies have shown little differences in functional outcomes among patients treated with CMC suspension arthroplasty procedures and arthrodesis [57], surgeons often prefer motion-preserving procedures for the CMC joint because the progression of the disease may later require MP or IP joint arthrodesis. Finally, compensatory hypermobility and degeneration at the adjacent MP joint make CMC joint arthrodesis a second line of treatment in patients who have rheumatoid arthritis.

Summary

Thumb involvement in rheumatoid arthritis is a common and important source of functional loss and disability. Proper understanding of the pathophysiology of the disease and the patient's activity level must be taken into consideration for appropriate planning in the surgical management of the disease. Conservative measures and less invasive surgical options can be used in patients who are in the early stages of disease. Arthrodesis or arthroplasty are used in cases of more severe joint involvement. The MP joint is usually the most affected by the disease and is best treated by arthrodesis. Activity level should also help guide the treating physician; low-demand patients or those who use finer dexterity are good candidates for arthroplasty, whereas arthrodesis can be used in high-demand, active patients.

References

[1] Alamanos Y, Voulgari PV, Drosos AA. Incidence and prevalence of rheumatoid arthritis, based on the 1987 American College of Rheumatology criteria: a systematic review. Semin Arthritis Rheum 2006;36(3):182–8.

[2] Terrono AL, Millender LH. The rheumatoid thumb. In: Strickland JW, editor. Master techniques in orthopaedic surgery: the hand. 1st edition. Philadelphia: Lippincott Williams and Wilkins; 1998. p. 439–46.

[3] Nalebuff EA. Diagnosis, classification and management of rheumatoid thumb deformities. Bull Hosp Joint Dis 1968;29:119–37.

[4] Terrono A, Nalebuff E, Philips C. The rheumatoid thumb. In: Hunter J, MacKin E, Callahan A, editors. Rehabilitation of the hand: surgery and therapy. 4th edition. St Louis (MO): Mosby; 1995. p. 1329–43.

[5] Millender LH, Nalebuff EA. Evaluation and treatment of early rheumatoid hand involvement. Orthop Clin North Am 1975;6:697–708.

[6] Rheumatoid Arthritis. American College of Rheumatology. Available at: http://www.rheumatology.org/public/factsheets/ra_new.asp?aud=pat. Accessed February 1, 2006.

[7] Rozental TD, Sculco TP. Intra-articular corticosteroids: an updated overview. Am J Orthop 2000;29:18–23.

[8] Ouellette EA. The rheumatoid hand: orthotics as preventative. Semin Arthritis Rheum 1991;21:65–72.

[9] O'Brien AV, Jones P, Mullis R, et al. Conservative hand therapy treatments in rheumatoid arthritis-a randomized controlled trial. Rheumatology 2006;45:577–83.

[10] Philips CA. Management of the patient with rheumatoid arthritis. The role of the hand therapist. Hand Clin 1989;5:291–309.

[11] Sagelback OE, Haga T. Surgical treatment of the rheumatoid thumb. Scand J Plast Reconstr Surg 1976;10:153–6.

[12] Nalebuff EA. Surgical treatment of tendon ruptures in the rheumatoid hand. Surg Clin North Am 1969;49:811–22.

[13] Terrono A, Millender L, Nalebuff EA. Boutonniere rheumatoid thumb deformity. J Hand Surg [Am] 1990;15:999–1003.

[14] Harrison SH, Ansell BM. Surgery of the rheumatoid thumb. Br J Plast Surg 1974;27:242–7.

[15] Manueddu CA, Bogoch ER, Hastings DE. Restoration of metacarpophalangeal extension of the thumb in inflammatory arthritis. J Hand Surg [Br] 1996;21:633–9.

[16] De Smet L, Van Loon J, Fabry G. Extensor indicis proprius to extensor pollicis longus transfer: results and complications. Acta Orthop Belg 1997;63:178–81.

[17] Inglis AE, Hamlin C, Senglemann RP, et al. Reconstruction of the metacarpophalangeal joint of the thumb in rheumatoid arthritis. J Bone Joint Surg Am 1972;54:704–12.

[18] Kessler I. A simplified technique to correct hyperextension of the metacarpophalangeal joint of the thumb. J Hand Surg [Am] 1979;61:903–5.

[19] Eaton RG, Floyd WE. Thumb metacarpophalangeal caspsulodesis: an adjunct procedure to basal joint arthroplasty for collapse deformity of the first ray. J Hand Surg [Am] 1988;13:449–53.

[20] Schuurman AH, Bos KE. Treatment of volar instability of the metacarpophalangeal joint of the thumb by volar capsulodesis. J Hand Surg [Br] 1993;18:346–9.

[21] Mannerfelt L, Norman O. Rupture of the extensor pollicis longus tendon after Colles' fractures and by rheumatoid arthritis. J Hand Surg [Br] 1990;15:49–50.

[22] Moore JR, Weiland AJ, Valdata L. Independent index extension after extensor indicis proprius transfer. J Hand Surg [Am] 1987;12:232–6.

[23] Terrono A, Millender L, Nalebuff EA. Boutonniere rheumatoid thumb deformity. J Hand Surg 1990;15A:999–1003.

[24] Stein AB, Terrono AL. The rheumatoid thumb. Hand Clin 1996;12(3):541–50.

[25] Mannerfelt L, Norman O. Attrition ruptures of flexor tendons in rheumatoid arthritis caused by bony spurs in the carpal tunnel. A clinical and radiologic study. J Bone Joint Surg Br 1969;51:270–7.

[26] Ertel AN. Flexor tendon ruptures in rheumatoid arthritis. Hand Clin 1988;13:860–6.

[27] Swanson A, Herndon J. Flexible (silicone) implant arthroplasty of the metacarpophalangeal joint of the thumb. J Bone Joint Surg Am 1977;59:362–8.

[28] Figgie MP, Inglis AE, Sobel M, et al. Metacarpalphalangeal joint arthroplasty of the rheumatoid thumb. J Hand Surg [Am] 1990;15:210–6.

[29] Flatt A, Ellison M. Restoration of rheumatoid finger joint function. J Bone Joint Surg Am 1972;54:1317–22.

[30] Blair W, Shurr D, Buckwalter J. Metacarpophalangeal joint implant arthroplasty with a silastic spacer. J Bone Joint Surg Am 1984;66:365–70.

[31] McGovern RM, Shin AY, Beckenbaugh RD, et al. Long-term results of cemented Steffee arthroplasty of the thumb metacarpophalangeal joint. J Hand Surg [Am] 2001;26:115–22.

[32] Bieber EJ, Weiland AJ, Volnec-Dowling S. Silicone rubber implant arthroplasty of the metacarpalphalangeal joints for rheumatoid arthritis. J Bone Joint Surg Am 1986;68:206–9.

[33] Murray PM. Current status of metacarpophalangeal arthroplasty and basilar joint arthroplasty of the thumb. Clin Plast Surg 1996;23:395–406.

[34] Swanson A, de Groot Swanson D, Watermeier J. Trapezium implant arthroplasty: long-term evaluation of 150 cases. J Hand Surg [Am] 1981;6:125–41.

[35] Smith RJ, Atkinson RE, Jupiter JB. Silicone synovitis of the wrist. J Hand Surg [Am] 1985;10:47–60.

[36] Peimer CA, Medige J, Eckert BS, et al. Reactive synovitis after silicone arthroplasty. J Hand Surg [Am] 1986;11:624–38.

[37] Creighton J, Steichen J, Strickland J. Long-term evaluation of silastic trapezial arthroplasty in patients with osteoarthritis. J Hand Surg [Am] 1991;16:510–9.

[38] Bezwada HP, Sauer ST, Hankins ST, et al. Long-term results of trapeziometacarpal silicone arthroplasty. J Hand Surg [Am] 2002;27(3):409–17.

[39] Eaton RG. Replacement of the trapezium for arthritis of the basal articulations: a new technique with stabilization by tenodesis. J Bone Joint Surg Am 1979;61(1):76–82.

[40] Adams B, Unsell R, McLaughlin P. Niebauer trapeziometacarpal arthroplasty. J Hand Surg [Am] 1990;15:487–92.

[41] Sotereanos DG, Taras J, Urbaniak JR. Niebauer trapeziometacarpal arthroplasty: a long-term follow-up. J Hand Surg [Am] 1993;18:560–4.

[42] Athwal GS, Chenkin J, King GJ, et al. Early failures with a spheric interposition arthroplasty of the thumb basal joint. J Hand Surg [Am] 2004;29:1080–4.

[43] Uchiyama S, Cooney WP, Niebur G, et al. Biomechanical analysis of the trapeziometacarpal joint after surface replacement arthroplasty. J Hand Surg [Am] 1999;24:483–90.

[44] Wacthl SW, Guggenheim PR, Senwald GR. Cemented and non-cemented replacements of the trapeziometacarpal joint. J Bone Joint Surg Br 1998;80(1):121–5.

[45] Burton RI, Pellegrini VD Jr. Surgical management of basal joint arthritis of the thumb. Part II. Ligament reconstruction with tendon interposition arthroplasty. J Hand Surg [Am] 1986;11:324–32.

[46] Tomaino MM, Pellegrini VD, Burton RI. Arthroplasty of the basal joint of the thumb. Long-term follow-up after ligament reconstruction with tendon interposition. J Bone Joint Surg Am 1995; 77:346–55.

[47] Weilby A. Tendon interposition arthroplasty of the first carpo-metacarpal joint. J Hand Surg [Br] 1988;13:421–5.

[48] Sigfusson R, Lundborg G. Abductor pollicis longus tendon arthroplasty for treatment of arthrosis in the first carpometacarpal joint. Scand J Plast Reconstr Surg Hand Surg 1991;25:73–7.

[49] Necking LE, Eiken O. ECRL-strip plasty for metacarpal base fixation after excision of the trapezium. Scand J Plast Reconstr Surg 1986;20: 229–33.

[50] Dell P, Brushart T, Smith R. Treatment of trapeziometacarpal arthritis: results of resection arthroplasty. J Hand Surg [Am] 1978;3:243–9.

[51] Ferlic DC, Turner BD, Clayton ML. Compression arthrodesis of the thumb. J Hand Surg [Am] 1983; 8:207–10.

[52] Carroll RE, Hill NA. Small joint arthrodesis in hand reconstruction. J Bone Joint Surg Am 1969;51: 1219–21.

[53] Katzman SS, Gibeault JD, Dickson K, et al. Use of a Herbert screw for interphalangeal joint arthrodesis. Clin Orthop 1993;296:127–32.

[54] Brutus JP, Palmer AK, Mosher JF, et al. Use of a headless compressive screw for distal interphalangeal joint arthrodesis in digits: clinical outcome and review of complications. J Hand Surg [Am] 2006; 31(1):85–9.

[55] Stanley JK, Smith EJ, Muirhead AG. Arthrodesis of the metacarpo-phalangeal joint of the thumb: a review of 42 cases. J Hand Surg [Br] 1989;14: 291–3.

[56] Nalebuff EA, Garrett J. Opera-glass hand in rheumatoid arthritis. J Hand Surg [Am] 1976;1: 210–20.

[57] Hartigan BJ, Stern PJ, Kiefhaber TR. Thumb carpometacarpal osteoarthritis: arthrodesis compared with ligament reconstruction and tendon interposition. J Bone Joint Surg Am 2001;83(10): 1470–8.

Index

Note: Page numbers of article titles are in **boldface** type.

0749-0712/08/$ - see front matter © 2008 Elsevier Inc. All rights reserved.
doi:10.1016/S0749-0712(08)00063-2

Moving?

Make sure your subscription moves with you!

To notify us of your new address, find your **Clinics Account Number** (located on your mailing label above your name), and contact customer service at:

E-mail: elspcs@elsevier.com

800-654-2452 (subscribers in the U.S. & Canada)
1-407-563-6020 (subscribers outside of the U.S. & Canada)

Fax number: 407-363-9661

Elsevier Periodicals Customer Service
6277 Sea Harbor Drive
Orlando, FL 32887-4800

*To ensure uninterrupted delivery of your subscription, please notify us at least 4 weeks in advance of move.